Study Guide for Ricci's

Essentials of Maternity, Newborn, and Women's Health Nursing

SECOND EDITION

Wolters Kluwer | Lippincott Williams & Wilkins
Health
Philadelphia · Baltimore · New York · London
Buenos Aires · Hong Kong · Sydney · Tokyo

Managing Editor: Annette Ferran
Senior Production Editor: Tom Gibbons
Director of Nursing Production: Helen Ewan
Senior Managing Editor/Production: Erika Kors
Manufacturing Coordinator: Karin Duffield
Compositor: Aptara

2nd Edition
Copyright © 2009 Wolters Kluwer Health | Lippincott Williams & Wilkins.

9 8 7 6 5 4 3

Printed in the United State of America

ISBN-13: 978-1-6054-7628-5

Care has been taken to confirm the accuracy of the information presented and to describe generally accepted practices. However, the authors, editors, and publisher are not responsible for errors or omissions or for any consequences from application of the information in this book and make no warranty, expressed or implied, with respect to the currency, completeness, or accuracy of the contents of the publication. Application of this information in a particular situation remains the professional responsibility of the practitioner; the clinical treatments described and recommended may not be considered absolute and universal recommendations.

The authors, editors, and publisher have exerted every effort to ensure that drug selection and dosage set forth in this text are in accordance with the current recommendations and practice at the time of publication. However, in view of ongoing research, changes in government regulations, and the constant flow of information relating to drug therapy and drug reactions, the reader is urged to check the package insert for each drug for any change in indications and dosage and for added warnings and precautions. This is particularly important when the recommended agent is a new or infrequently employed drug.

Some drugs and medical devices presented in this publication have Food and Drug Administration (FDA) clearance for limited use in restricted research settings. It is the responsibility of the health care provider to ascertain the FDA status of each drug or device planned for use in his or her clinical practice.

Preface

This Study Guide was developed by the Instructional Design firm of LearningMate and reviewed by Kathleen Beebe, RNC, PhD, Jo Anne Kirk, MSN, RN, and Susan Miovech, PhD, RNC, to accompany *Essentials of Maternity, Newborn, and Women's Health Nursing,* 2nd edition, by Susan Scott Ricci. The Study Guide is designed to help you practice and retain the knowledge you have gained from the textbook, and it is structured to integrate that knowledge and give you a basis for applying it in your nursing practice. The following types of exercises are provided in each chapter of the Study Guide.

ASSESSING YOUR UNDERSTANDING

The first section of each Study Guide chapter concentrates on the basic information of the textbook chapter and helps you to remember key concepts, vocabulary, and principles.

- *Fill in the Blanks*

Fill in the blank exercises test important chapter information, encouraging you to recall key points.

- *Labeling*

Labeling exercises are used where you need to remember certain visual representations of the concepts presented in the textbook.

- *Match the Following*

Matching questions test your knowledge of the definition of key terms.

- *Sequencing*

Sequencing exercises ask you to remember particular sequences or orders, for example, testing processes and prioritizing nursing actions.

- *Short Answers*

Short answer questions cover facts, concepts, procedures, and principles of the chapter. These questions ask you to recall information as well as demonstrate your comprehension of the information.

APPLYING YOUR KNOWLEDGE

The second section of each Study Guide chapter consists of case study–based exercises that ask you to begin to apply the knowledge you've gained from the textbook chapter and reinforced in the first section of the Study Guide chapter. A case study scenario based on the chapter's content is presented, and then you are asked to answer some questions, in writing, related to the case study. The questions cover the following areas:

- Assessment
- Planning Nursing Care
- Communication
- Reflection

PRACTICING FOR NCLEX

The third and final section of the Study Chapters helps you practice NCLEX-style questions while further reinforcing the knowledge you have been gaining and testing for yourself through the textbook chapter and the first two sections of the study guide chapter. In keeping with the NCLEX, the questions presented are multiple-choice and scenario-based, asking you to reflect, consider, and apply what you know and to choose the best answer out of those offered.

ANSWER KEYS

The answers for all of the exercises and questions in the Study Guide are provided at the back of the book, so you can assess your own learning as you complete each chapter.

We hope you will find this Study Guide to be helpful and enjoyable, and we wish you every success in your studies toward becoming a nurse.

The Publishers

Contents

CHAPTER 1

Perspectives on Maternal, Newborn, and Women's Health Care

SECTION I: LEARNING OBJECTIVES

1. Identify the key milestones in the evolution of maternal, newborn, and women's health nursing.

2. Describe the major components, concepts, and influences associated with the nursing management of women and their families.

3. Compare the past definitions of health and illness to the current definitions.

4. Identify the factors that affect maternal, newborn, and women's health.

5. Evaluate how society and culture can influence the health of women and their families.

6. Appraise the health care barriers affecting women and their families.

7. Discuss the ethical and legal issues that may arise when caring for women and their families.

SECTION II: ASSESSING YOUR UNDERSTANDING

Activity A *Fill in the blanks.*

1. A _____ is a lay birth assistant who provides quality emotional, physical, and educational support to the woman and family during childbirth and the postpartum period.

2. _____ fetal surgery is a procedure that involves opening the uterus during pregnancy, performing a surgery, and replacing the fetus in the uterus.

3. The use of oral contraceptives makes a woman susceptible to _____ cancer.

4. The _____ is considered the basic social unit.

5. Under certain conditions, a minor can be considered _____ and can make health care decisions independently of parents.

6. Overall plans in the health care delivery system improve access to preventive services, but may limit the access to _____ care which greatly impacts women and children with chronic or long-term illnesses.

7. The process of increasing desirable behavior and decreasing or eliminating undesirable behavior is known as _____.

8. The ability to apply knowledge about a client's culture to adapt his or her health care accordingly is known as cultural _____.

9. With the emphasis on reducing costs and preventive care and services, _____ guidance and education by nurses has become ever more important.

10. _____ is the measure of prevalence of a specific illness in a population at a particular time.

Match the cultural group in column A with the proper belief or practice affecting maternal and infant health in column B.

Column A

_____ **1.** Asian-Americans

_____ **2.** African-Americans

_____ **3.** Arab-Americans

_____ **4.** Native-Americans

_____ **5.** Hispanics

Column B

a. Mother's legs brought together after birth of newborn to prevent air from entering uterus

b. Wrapping of newborn's stomach at birth to prevent cold or wind from entering baby's body

c. Newborn not given colostrums

d. Quiet, stoic appearance of woman during labor

e. Liberal use of oil on newborn's and infant's scalp and skin

Using the boxes provided below, put the following characteristic approaches in the evolution of maternal and newborn nursing in the proper chronological order.

1.

  a. The assistance of certified nurse midwives and doulas grew in popularity as a choice in childbirth

  b. "Granny midwives" handled the normal birthing process for most women; infant and maternal mortality rates were high.

  c. "Natural childbirth" practices advocating birth without medication and focusing on relaxation techniques were introduced.

  d. Physicians attended about half the births, with midwives caring for women who could not afford a doctor.

Briefly answer the following.

1. What are the risk factors the nurse should monitor for in women that could lead to CVD?

_____

_____

_____

2. What are the components of case management?

_____

_____

_____

3. What are the risk factors for breast cancer in women?

_____

_____

_____

4. What is evidence-based nursing practice?

_____

_____

_____

5. What is maternal mortality rate?

_____

_____

_____

6. What are the predictors of infant mortality?

_____

_____

_____

SECTION III: APPLYING YOUR KNOWLEDGE

Activity E *Consider this scenario and answer the questions.*

A couple in their late 20s are expecting their first child. They are touring the labor and delivery suite at the hospital they have chosen for the birth. The nurse who is conducting the tour refers to giving "family centered care" and using "evidence-based nursing" on their unit.

1. During the question and answer period, the couple ask what "family-centered care" is. How would the nurse respond to this couple's question?

   _____

   _____

   _____

2. The couple then asks what the nurse means by "evidence-based nursing" and how that affects the two of them and their newborn. What is the nurse's best response?

   _____

   _____

   _____

SECTION IV: PRACTICING FOR NCLEX

Activity F *Answer the following questions.*

1. A female client who has just given birth has been reading health reports and is alarmed at the high rate of infant mortality. She seems anxious about the health of her child and wants to know ways to keep her baby from getting an infection. Which of the following instructions should the nurse offer?

   a. Place the infant on his or her back to sleep
   b. Breastfeed the infant
   c. Feed the infant foods high in starch
   d. Feed the infant liquids frequently

2. A group of nurses are running a campaign initiated by the Maternal and Child Health Bureau to educate women about better maternal and infant care. Which of the following measures should they advocate for the prevention of neural defects in infants?

   a. Take folic acid supplements
   b. Take vitamin E supplements
   c. Perform mild exercises during pregnancy
   d. Regularly eat citrus fruits during pregnancy

3. A nurse is caring for a client who wishes to undergo an abortion. The nurse has concerns because abortion is against her personal convictions, and this is interfering with her professional duty. Which of the following should the nurse do to follow ANA's code of ethics for nurses?

   a. Provide emotional support to the client while caring for her
   b. Not allow her personal convictions to interfere with her profession
   c. Involve the client's family in convincing the client against an abortion
   d. Make arrangements for alternate care providers

4. A female client who has just given birth arrives in a health care facility wanting to know of ways to prevent sudden infant death syndrome (SIDS). Which of the following instructions should the nurse provide?

   a. Drape the infant in warm clothes
   b. Feed a mixture of salts, sugar, and water
   c. Provide very soft bedding
   d. Place the infant on his or her back to sleep

5. A nurse is caring for a critically ill female client who has recently been diagnosed with advanced lung cancer. Which of the following reasons could have contributed to the late detection and diagnosis?

   a. Women have a stronger resistance against lung cancer
   b. Lung cancer has no early symptoms
   c. Lung cancer is considered more deadly in men than women
   d. Lung cancer is more challenging to diagnose in women than men

6. It is important to be able to measure the health status of a group of people or a nation so that the number of people who die prematurely will decrease over time. How does the United States measure the health status of its people?

    a. Tracks the incidence of violent crime

    b. Examines health disparities between ethnic groups

    c. Examines mortality and morbidity data

    d. Identifies specific national health goals related to maternal and infant health

7. The nurse is caring for an Arab-American woman. Which approach would be most successful?

    a. Inquiring about folk remedies used

    b. Coordinating care through the client's mother

    c. Dealing exclusively with the husband

    d. Promoting preventive health care

8. The nurse is caring for a client with end-stage breast cancer. When she takes chemotherapy medication into the client's room, the client states, "I'm too tired to fight any more. I don't want any more medication that may prolong my life." The client's husband is at the bedside and states, "No! You have to give my wife her medication. I can't let her go." What action by the nurse is most appropriate?

    a. Giving the medication

    b. Explaining to the husband that his wife has the right to refuse medication and care

    c. Encouraging the client to heed her husband's wishes

    d. Stating that she has to give the medication unless the doctor orders the medication stopped

9. A client is getting divorced and wants to be sure that her soon-to-be ex-husband cannot have access to her medical information. Which would be the best instruction for the nurse to give the client?

    a. "Don't worry about things like that, you have too much else to worry about right now."

    b. "Husbands always have access to their wife's health records."

    c. "We have to give him access to your records in case they impact your divorce proceedings."

    d. "You have the right to say who can see your health records and who cannot."

10. A nurse is caring for a 31-year-old pregnant female client who is subjected to abuse by her partner. The client has developed a feeling of hopelessness and does not feel confident in dealing with the situation at home, which makes her feel suicidal. Which of the following nursing interventions should the nurse offer to help the client deal with her situation?

    a. Counsel the client's partner to refrain from subjecting his partner to abuse

    b. Help the client understand the legal impact of her situation to protect her

    c. Provide emotional support to empower the client to help herself

    d. Introduce the client to a women's rights group

CHAPTER 2

Family-Centered Community-Based Care

SECTION I: LEARNING OBJECTIVES

1. Examine the major components and key elements of family-centered home health care.

2. Explain the reasons for the increased emphasis on community-based care.

3. Differentiate community-based nursing from nursing in acute care settings.

4. Explain the different levels of prevention in community-based nursing, providing examples of each.

5. Give examples of cultural issues that may be faced when providing community-based nursing.

6. Provide culturally competent care to women and their families.

7. Identify the variety of settings where community-based care can be provided to women and their families.

8. Outline the various roles and functions assumed by the community health nurse.

9. Demonstrate the ability to use excellent therapeutic communication skills when interacting with women and their families.

10. Explain the process of health teaching as it relates to women and their families.

11. Examine the importance of discharge planning and case management in providing community-based care.

SECTION II: ASSESSING YOUR UNDERSTANDING

Activity A *Fill in the blanks.*

1. _____ communication, also referred to as body language, includes attending to others and active listening.

2. _____ management focuses on coordinating health care services while balancing quality and cost outcomes.

3. _____ may be defined as a "specific group of people, often living in a defined geographical area, who share a common culture, values, and norms.

4. _____ clinics offer a community-based site for the childbearing family to access services.

5. Primary _____ involves avoiding the disease or condition before it occurs through health promotion activities, environmental protection, and specific protection against disease or injury.

6. Practicing true _____ care may empower the family, strengthen family resources, and help the woman or child feel more secure throughout the process.

7. Cultural _____ is defined as the knowledge, willingness, and ability to adapt health care to enhance its acceptability to and effectiveness with patients from diverse cultures.

8. Cultural _____ involve participating in cross-cultural interactions with people from culturally diverse backgrounds.

9. _____ literacy is the ability to read, understand and use health care information.

10. Medically _____ infants have medically complex needs that require skilled nursing interventions.

Activity B *Consider the following figure.*

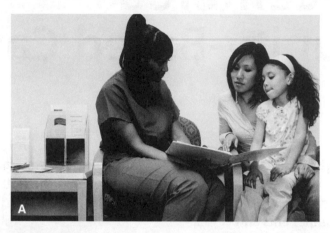

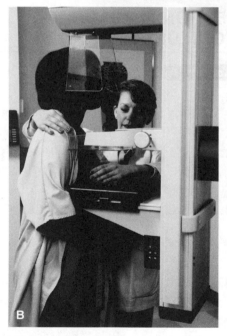

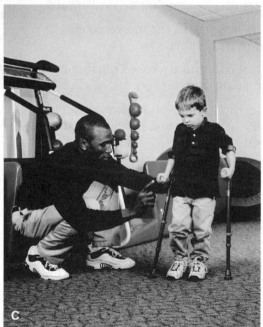

1. What does the figure depict?

_____

_____

Activity C *Match the health care facilities in Column A with their services in Column B.*

Column A

_____ **1.** Counseling centers

_____ **2.** Wellness centers

_____ **3.** Wholeness healing centers

_____ **4.** Educational centers

Column B

a. Provide women's health lectures, instruction on breast self-examinations and Pap smears, and computers for research

b. Provide acupuncture, aromatherapy, and herbal remedies

c. Offer stress reduction techniques

d. Offer various support groups

Activity D *Given below, in random order, are steps of patient and family education. Arrange them in the correct sequence, using the boxes below.*

1.

a. Intervening to enhance learning

b. Planning education

c. Evaluating learning

d. Documenting teaching and learning

e. Assessing teaching and learning needs

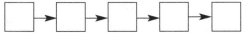

Activity E *Briefly answer the following.*

1. What techniques can the nurse use to enhance learning?

_____

_____

_____

2. What are the four main purposes of nursing documentation?

_____

_____

_____

3. What are the duties of a nurse in an outpatient clinic?

_____

_____

_____

4. What do discharge planning and case management contribute to in the community setting?

_____

_____

_____

5. What are the factors that have influenced an increased emphasis on health promotion and illness prevention?

_____

_____

_____

6. What is a birthing center?

_____

_____

_____

SECTION III: APPLYING YOUR KNOWLEDGE

Activity F *Consider the scenario and answer the questions.*

By the year 2050, people of African, Asian, and Latino backgrounds will make up one-half of the American population. This growing diversity has strong implications for the provision of health care.

1. A nurse is employed in a clinic that provides prenatal services to a multicultural community predominated by African and Latino families. How should the nurse adapt to different cultural beliefs and practices?

_____

_____

_____

2. List examples of cultural characteristics that would be important for a nurse to understand.

_____

_____

_____

3. What activities would help assure that a nurse delivers culturally competent nursing care to diverse families?

_____

_____

_____

SECTION IV: PRACTICING FOR NCLEX

Activity G   *Answer the following questions.*

1. Nurses in community care settings spend more time in management and supervisory roles than their counterparts in the acute care setting. Which of the following activities is part of case management?
   a. Helping a grandmother to learn a procedure
   b. Assessing the sanitary conditions of the home
   c. Establishing eligibility for a Medicaid waiver
   d. Scheduling speech and respiratory therapy services

2. What is a key element when providing family-centered care?
   a. Communicating specific health information
   b. Being in control of the way care is given
   c. Giving only the health information that is absolutely necessary while providing care to the client and their family.
   d. Avoid cultural issues by providing care in a standardized fashion

3. The nurse is educating the family of a two-day-old Chinese boy with myelomeningocele about the disorder and its treatment. Which of the following actions, involving an interpreter, can jeopardize the family's trust?
   a. Allowing too little appointment time for the translation
   b. Using a person who is not a professional interpreter

   c. Asking the interpreter questions not meant for the family
   d. Using a relative to communicate with the parents

4. The nurse is striving to form a partnership with the family of a medically fragile child being cared for at home. Which of the following activities is part of family-centered home care?
   a. Recognizing unique family strengths
   b. Ensuring a safe, nurturing environment
   c. Managing information given to parents
   d. Correcting inadequate coping methods

5. Nurses play important roles in a variety of community settings. Which of the following goals is common to all community settings?
   a. Remove or minimize health barriers to learning
   b. Promote the health of a specific group of clients
   c. Determine initially the type of care a client needs
   d. Ensure the health and well-being of women and their families

6. A nurse is assigned to take care of a high-risk newborn in the home environment after discharge. Which of the following conditions should the nurse monitor for in the infant?
   a. Anencephaly
   b. Hydrocephalus
   c. Fetal distress syndrome
   d. Spina bifida

7. A pregnant client arrives at the maternity clinic for a routine check-up. The client has been reading books on pregnancy and wants to know ways to prevent the incidence of neural tube defects (NTDs) in her fetus. Which of the following should the nurse offer the client to prevent the occurrence of NTDs?
   a. Take vitamin E supplements
   b. Take folic acid supplements
   c. Consume legumes frequently
   d. Consume citrus fruits frequently

8. A nurse has to address a group of women on the issue of women's health during their reproductive years. Which of the following reasons does the nurse provide regarding the need for comprehensive, community-centered care to women during their reproductive years?

   a. Women have more health problems during their reproductive years

   b. Women are more susceptible to stress during their reproductive years

   c. Women's immune system weakens immediately after birth

   d. Women's health care needs change with their reproductive goals

9. The nurse has to prepare a discharge plan as a part of her postpartum care of a client, whom she is caring for in a home-based setting. Which of the following aspects of care should the nurse include in her postpartum care in this environment?

   a. Provide the client with self-help books about infant care

   b. Monitor the physical and emotional well-being of family members

   c. Recognize infant needs in the discharge plan

   d. Identify developing complications in the infant

10. A nurse is caring for a Turkish client. The nurse understands that there could be major cultural differences between her and her client. What could be the consequence of a nurse assigning a client to a staff member who is of the same culture as the client?

    a. Lead to stereotyping

    b. Ensure better care and understanding

    c. Help in assessing client's culture

    d. Help build better nurse–client relationship

Anatomy and Physiology of the Reproductive System

SECTION I: LEARNING OBJECTIVES

1. Define the key terms utilized in this chapter.

2. Explain the structure and function of the major external and internal female genital organs.

3. Outline the phases of the menstrual cycle, dominant hormones involved, and changes taking place in each phase.

4. Classify external and internal male reproductive structures and the function of each in hormonal regulation.

SECTION II: ASSESSING YOUR UNDERSTANDING

Activity A *Fill in the blanks.*

1. The vagina is a tubular, fibromuscular organ lined with mucous membrane that lies in a series of transverse folds called _____.

2. _____ stimulates the production of milk within a few days after childbirth.

3. The _____, which lies against the testes, is a coiled tube almost 20 feet long that collects sperm from the testes and provides the space and environment for sperm to mature.

4. In the male, the _____ is the terminal duct of the reproductive and urinary systems, serving as a passageway for semen and urine.

5. The _____ is the mucosal layer that lines the uterine cavity in nonpregnant women.

6. _____ glands, located on either side of the female urethral opening, secrete a small amount of mucus to keep the opening moist and lubricated for the passage of urine.

7. The incision made into the perineal tissue to provide more space for the presenting part of the delivering fetus is called an _____.

8. In the male, the _____ gland lies just under the bladder in the pelvis and surrounds the middle portion of the urethra.

9. The _____ is a pear-shaped muscular organ at the top of the vagina.

10. The _____ is the thin-skinned sac that surrounds and protects the testes.

Activity B *Consider the following figures.*

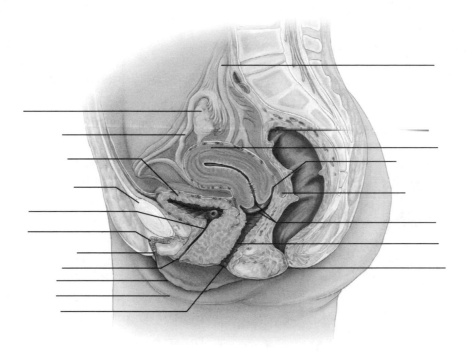

1. a. Identify and label the figure.

_____

_____

b. What are the various parts and their functions?

_____

_____

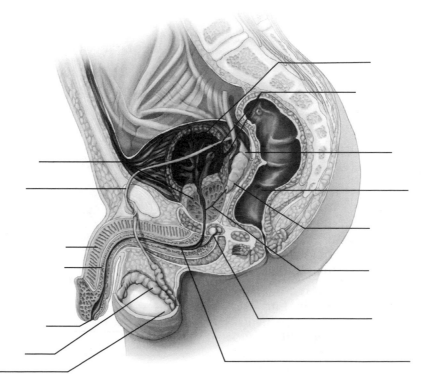

2. a. Identify and label the figure.

_____

_____

b. What are the various parts and their functions?

_____

_____

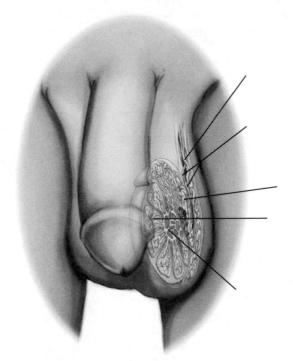

3. Identify and label the figure.

_____

_____

Column A

____ **1.** Gonadotropin-Releasing Hormone (GnRH)

____ **2.** Follicle-Stimulating Hormone (FSH)

____ **3.** Luteinizing Hormone (LH)

____ **4.** Estrogen

____ **5.** Progesterone

Column B

a. It maintains the uterine decidual lining and reduces uterine contractions, allowing pregnancy to be maintained.

b. It is required for the final maturation of preovulatory follicles and luteinization of the ruptured follicle.

c. It is primarily responsible for the maturation of the ovarian follicle.

d. It inhibits FSH production and stimulates LH production.

e. It induces the release of FSH and LH to assist with ovulation.

1. Given below, in random order, are steps occurring during the endometrial cycle. Arrange them in the correct sequence.

a. The endometrium becomes thickened and more vascular and glandular.

b. Cervical mucus becomes thin, clear, stretchy, and more alkaline.

c. The spiral arteries rupture, releasing blood into the uterus.

d. The ischemia leads to shedding of the endometrium down to the basal layer.

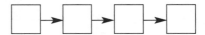

2. Given below, in random order, are pubertal events. Arrange them in the correct sequence.

a. Growth spurt

b. Appearance of pubic and then axillary hair

c. Development of breast buds

d. Onset of menstruation

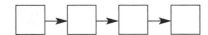

1. What is the vulva?

_____

_____

_____

2. What is colostrum?

_____

_____

_____

3. What are the physical changes observed in women during their perimenopausal years?

_____

_____

_____

4. What is the role of the nurse when caring for menopausal women?

_____

_____

_____

5. What is the function of the testes?

_____

_____

_____

6. What is the function of the bulbourethral, or Cowper's, glands?

_____

_____

_____

SECTION III: APPLYING YOUR KNOWLEDGE

Activity F *Consider this scenario and answer the questions.*

Susan is a 14-year-old high school student who came to the school nurse's office because she had her first period. She has received health education information in class, but Susan has many questions about her body. She asks the school nurse a lot of questions.

a. Describe what a nurse should teach Susan about the changes in her body and menstruation.

_____

_____

_____

b. Describe the nurse's response when Susan asks how long her cycles will last.

_____

_____

_____

SECTION IV: PRACTICING FOR NCLEX

Activity G *Answer the following questions.*

1. A client is trying to have a baby and wants to know the best time to have intercourse to increase the chances of pregnancy. Which of the following is the ideal time for intercourse, to help her chances of conceiving?

   a. A week after ovulation

   b. One or two days before ovulation

   c. Anytime after ovulation

   d. Anytime during the week before ovulation

2. Which of the following organs is responsible for providing lubrication during intercourse?

   a. Endocrine glands

   b. Pituitary glands

   c. Skene's glands

   d. Bartholin's glands

3. Which of the following is the mucosal layer that lines the uterine cavity in nonpregnant women?

   a. Endometrium

   b. Fundus

   c. Mons pubis

   d. Clitoris

4. A nurse is caring for a client who has given birth. The client reports that her breast milk is dark yellow. Which of the following information should the nurse give to the client regarding the situation?

   a. Modify diet to reduce excess fat intake

   b. The yellow fluid is colostrum and is rich in maternal antibodies

   c. Breastfeeding should be avoided until the breast milk becomes normal

   d. Completely stop breastfeeding and use formula instead

5. A client complains of pain on one side of the abdomen. On further questioning, the nurse discovers that the pain occurs regularly around two weeks before menstruation. The client has not missed a period, and she exercises regularly. Which of the following is the most likely cause of the pain?

   a. Early signs of pregnancy
   b. Irregular menstruation cycle
   c. Pain during ovulation
   d. Exercising regularly

6. A client asks the nurse how she would know if ovulation has occurred. Which of the following is a sign of ovulation that the nurse should inform the client about?

   a. Pain in the vaginal area
   b. Rise in temperature by 0.5–1°F
   c. Uneasiness or sickness
   d. Lack of sleep

7. A nurse is assessing a 45-year-old client. The client asks for information regarding the changes that are most likely to occur with menopause. Which of the following should the nurse tell the client?

   a. Uterus tilts backward
   b. Uterus shrinks and gradually atrophies
   c. Cervical muscle content increases
   d. Outer layer of the cervix becomes rough

8. Which of the following hormones is called the hormone of pregnancy because it reduces uterine contractions during pregnancy?

   a. Luteinizing hormone
   b. Estrogen
   c. Follicle-stimulating hormone
   d. Progesterone

9. During cold conditions, how does the body react to maintain scrotal temperature?

   a. Cremaster muscles relax
   b. Frequency of urination increases
   c. Scrotum is pulled closer to the body
   d. Increase in blood flow to genital area

10. A nurse is screening an elderly client for prostate cancer. What are the effects of aging on the prostate gland?

    a. Prostate gland enlarges with age
    b. Production of semen stops
    c. Prostate gland stops functioning
    d. Prostate gland causes painful erection

11. Which of the following organs provides the space and environment for sperm cells to mature?

    a. Vas deferens
    b. Epididymis
    c. Testes
    d. Cowper's glands

12. A nurse is explaining the menstrual cycle to a 12-year-old client who has experienced menarche. Which of the following should the nurse tell the client?

    a. An average cycle length is about 15 to 20 days
    b. Ovary contains 400,000 follicles at birth
    c. Duration of the flow is about 3 to 7 days
    d. Blood loss averages 120 to 150 mL

13. A nurse is providing information regarding ovulation to a couple who want to have a baby. Which of the following should the nurse tell the clients?

    a. Ovulation takes place 10 days before menstruation
    b. The lifespan of the ovum is only about 48 hours
    c. At ovulation, a mature follicle ruptures, releasing an ovum
    d. When ovulation occurs, there is a rise in estrogen

14. Which of the following hormones is secreted from the hypothalamus in a pulsatile manner throughout the reproductive cycle?

    a. Follicle-stimulating hormone
    b. Gonadotropin-releasing hormone
    c. Luteinizing hormone
    d. Estrogen

CHAPTER 4

Common Reproductive Issues

SECTION I: LEARNING OBJECTIVES

1. Define the key terms utilized in this chapter.

2. Examine common reproductive concerns in terms of symptoms, diagnostic tests, and appropriate interventions.

3. Identify risk factors and outline appropriate client education needed in common reproductive disorders.

4. Compare and contrast the various contraceptive methods available and their overall effectiveness.

5. Explain the physiologic and psychological aspects of menopause.

6. Delineate the nursing management needed for women experiencing common reproductive disorders.

SECTION II: ASSESSING YOUR UNDERSTANDING

Activity A *Fill in the blanks.*

1. _____ involves the in-growth of the endometrium into the uterine musculature.

2. Primary dysmenorrhea is caused by increased _____ production by the endometrium in an ovulatory cycle.

3. _____ is the direct visualization of the internal organs with a lighted instrument inserted through an abdominal incision.

4. During _____, the ovary begins to sputter, producing irregular and missed periods and an occasional hot flash.

5. Male sterilization is accomplished with a surgical procedure known as a _____.

6. In a _____ abortion, the woman takes certain medications to induce a miscarriage to remove the products of conception.

7. _____ is a condition in which bone mass declines to such an extent that fractures occur with minimal trauma.

8. At the onset of ovulation, cervical mucus that is more abundant, clear, slippery, and smooth is known as _____ mucus.

9. The _____ body temperature refers to the lowest body temperature and is reached upon awakening.

10. Oral contraceptives, called _____, contain only progestin and work primarily by thickening the cervical mucus to prevent penetration of the sperm and make the endometrium unfavorable for implantation.

Activity B *Consider the following figures.*

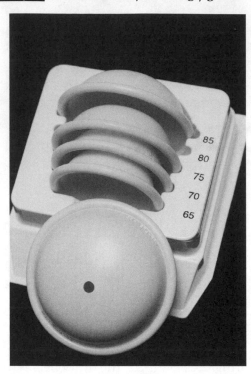

1. What is the purpose of this device?

_____

_____

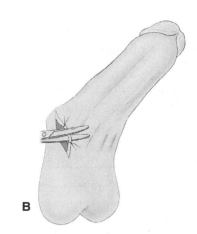

B

2. a. What is being done in this procedure?

_____

_____

b. What is the outcome of this procedure?

_____

_____

Activity C *Match the terms in Column A with the definitions in Column B.*

Column A

_____ **1.** Amenorrhea

_____ **2.** Dysmenorrhea

_____ **3.** Metrorrhagia

_____ **4.** Menometrorrhagia

_____ **5.** Oligomenorrhea

Column B

a. Bleeding between periods

b. Bleeding occurring at intervals of more than 35 days

c. Absence of menses during the reproductive years

d. Difficult or painful or abnormal menstruation

e. Heavy bleeding occurring at irregular intervals, with flow lasting more than 7 days

Activity D *Put the steps in correct sequence by writing the letters in the boxes provided below.*

1. Given below, in random order, are steps occurring during diaphragm insertion. Write the correct sequence.

a. Hold the diaphragm between the thumb and fingers and compress it to form a "figure-eight" shape.

b. Place a tablespoon of spermicidal jelly or cream in the dome and around the rim of the diaphragm.

c. Select the position that is most comfortable for insertion.

d. Tuck the front rim of the diaphragm behind the pubic bone so that the rubber hugs the front wall of the vagina.

e. Insert the diaphragm into the vagina, directing it downward as far as it will go.

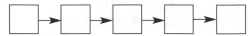

2. Given below, in random order, are steps occurring during cervical cap insertion. Write the correct sequence.

a. Pinch the sides of the cervical cap together.

b. Use one finger to feel around the entire circumference to make sure there are no gaps between the cap rim and the cervix.

c. Pinch the cap dome and tug gently to check for evidence of suction.

d. Insert the cervical cap into the vagina, and place over the cervix.

e. Compress the cervical cap dome.

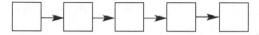

Activity E *Briefly answer the following.*

1. What are the common laboratory tests ordered to determine the cause of amenorrhea?

_____

_____

_____

2. What is menopause?

_____

_____

_____

3. What are the risk factors associated with endometriosis?

_____

_____

_____

4. What is infertility?

_____

_____

_____

5. What is the Two-Day Method for contraception?

_____

_____

_____

6. What are intrauterine systems?

_____

_____

_____

SECTION III: APPLYING YOUR KNOWLEDGE

Activity F *Consider this scenario and answer the questions.*

Alexa is a 14-year-old lacrosse player who has been training vigorously for selection on her high school team. Alexa comes to the health care provider's office to have her health forms for school completed. The office nurse takes her history, and the client describes that she has been experiencing amenorrhea.

1. How should the nurse describe "primary amenorrhea" to Alexa?

_____

_____

_____

2. State the causes of "primary amenorrhea" that may be related to Alexa.

_____

_____

_____

3. What treatments may be considered for Alexa?

_____

_____

_____

4. What counseling and education should the nurse provide for Alexa at this visit?

_____

_____

_____

SECTION IV: PRACTICING FOR NCLEX

Activity G *Answer the following questions.*

1. The nurse is assessing a client for amenorrhea. Which of the following should the nurse document as evidence of androgen excess secondary to a tumor?

a. Reduced subcutaneous fat

b. Hypothermia

c. Irregular heart rate and pulse

d. Facial hair and acne

2. A nurse is teaching a female client about fertility awareness as a method of contraception. Which of the following should the nurse mention as an assumption for this method?

a. Sperm can live up to 24 hours after intercourse

b. The "unsafe period" is approximately 6 days

c. The exact time of ovulation can be determined

d. The "safe period" is 3 days after ovulation

3. The nurse is instructing a client with dysmenorrhea on how to manage her symptoms. Which of the following should the nurse include in the teaching plan? Select all that apply.

a. Increase intake of salty foods

b. Increase water consumption

c. Avoid keeping legs elevated while lying down

d. Use heating pads or take warm baths

e. Increase exercise and physical activity

4. A client is to be examined for the presence and extent of endometriosis. Which of the following tests should the nurse prepare the client for?

a. Tissue biopsy

b. Hysterosalpingogram

c. Clomiphene citrate challenge test

d. Laparoscopy

5. A couple is being assessed for infertility. The male partner is required to collect a semen sample for analysis. What instruction should the nurse give him?

a. Abstain from sexual activity for 10 hours before collecting the sample

b. Avoid strenuous activity for 24 hours before collecting the sample

c. Collect a specimen by ejaculating into a condom or plastic bag

d. Deliver sample for analysis within 1 to 2 hours after ejaculation

6. A client needs additional information about the cervical mucus ovulation method after having read about it in a magazine. She asks the nurse about cervical changes during ovulation. Which of the following should the nurse inform the client about?

a. Cervical os is slightly closed

b. Cervical mucus is dry and thick

c. Cervix is high or deep in the vagina

d. Cervical mucus breaks when stretched

7. A female client has undergone a clomiphene citrate challenge test. The FSH level is 16.5. What should the nurse tell this client?

a. "This is a good result; we just need to chart your cycle."

b. "I'm sorry, but adoption seems to be your only option."

c. "You might want to consider the option of using donor eggs."

d. "Artificial insemination might be a solution to your problems."

8. A client has been following the conventional 28-day regimen for contraception. She is now considering switching to an extended Oral Contraceptive (OC) regimen. She is seeking information about specific safety precautions. Which of the following is true for the extended OC regimen?

a. It is not as effective as the conventional regimen

b. It prevents pregnancy for three months at a time

c. It carries the same safety profile as the 28-day regimen

d. It does not ensure restoration of fertility if discontinued

9. A 30-year-old client would like to try using basal body temperature (BBT) as a fertility awareness method. Which of the following instructions should the nurse provide the client?

a. Avoid unprotected intercourse until BBT has been elevated for six days

b. Avoid using other fertility awareness methods along with BBT

c. Use the axillary method of taking the temperature

d. Take temperature before rising and record it on a chart

10. A client who is not well-educated has approached the nurse for information about contraception. She indicates that she is not comfortable about using any barrier methods and would like the option of regaining fertility after a couple of years. Which of the following methods should the nurse suggest to this client?

a. Basal body temperature

b. Coitus interruptus

c. Lactational amenorrhea method

d. CycleBeads or Depo-Provera

11. A client would like some information about the use of a cervical cap. Which of the following should the nurse include in the teaching plan of this client? Select all that apply.

a. Inspect the cervical cap prior to insertion

b. Apply spermicide to the rim of the cervical cap

c. Wait for 30 minutes after insertion before engaging in intercourse

d. Remove the cervical cap immediately after intercourse

e. Do not use the cervical cap during menses

12. A healthy 28-year-old female client who has a sedentary lifestyle and is a chain smoker is seeking information about contraception. The nurse informs this client of the various options available and the benefits and the risks of each. Which of the following should the nurse recognize as contraindicated in the case of this client?

a. The Lunelle injection or Depo-Provera

b. Combination oral contraceptives

c. A copper intrauterine device

d. Implantable contraceptives

13. A client in her second trimester of pregnancy asks the nurse for information regarding certain oral medications to induce a miscarriage. What information should this client be given about such medications?

a. They are available only in the form of suppositories

b. They can be taken only in the first trimester

c. They present a high risk of respiratory failure

d. They are considered a permanent end to fertility

14. A client reports that she has multiple sex partners and has a lengthy history of various pelvic infections. She would like to know if there is any temporary contraceptive method that would suit her condition. Which of the following should the nurse suggest for this client?

a. Intrauterine device

b. Condoms

c. Oral contraceptives

d. Tubal ligation

15. When caring for a client with reproductive issues, the nurse is required to clear up misconceptions. This enables new learning to take hold and a better client response to whichever methods are explored and ultimately selected. Which of the following are misconceptions that the nurse needs to clear up? Select all that apply.

a. Breastfeeding does not protect against pregnancy

b. Taking birth control pills protects against STIs

c. Douching after sex will prevent pregnancy

d. Pregnancy can occur during menses

e. Irregular menstruation prevents pregnancy

16. A 52-year-old client is seeking treatment for menopause. She is not very active and has a history of cardiac problems. Which of the following therapy options should the nurse recognize as contraindicated for this client?

a. Long-term hormone replacement therapy

b. Selective estrogen receptor modulators

c. Lipid-lowering agents

d. Bisphosphonates

17. A 49-year-old client undergoing menopause complains to the nurse of loss of lubrication during intercourse, which she feels is hampering her sex life. Which of the following responses is appropriate for the nurse?

a. "Don't worry! This is a normal process of aging."

b. "Have you considered contacting a support group for women your age?"

c. "You can manage the condition by using OTC moisturizers or lubricants."

d. "All you need is a positive outlook and a supportive partner."

18. A couple is interested in seeking treatment for infertility. Which of the following should the nurse ensure in the initial stage?

    a. The couple is aware of the risks and benefits of treatments

    b. The couple has access to all the required medical facilities

    c. The couple is financially sound and can handle the treatment costs

    d. The couple's emotional distress level is not unusually high

19. A client has opted to use an intrauterine device for contraception. Which of the following effects of the device on monthly periods should the nurse inform the client about?

    a. Periods become lighter

    b. Periods become more painful

    c. Periods become longer

    d. Periods reduce in number

20. A 30-year-old client tells the nurse that she would like to use a contraceptive sponge but does not know enough about its use and whether it will protect her against sexually transmitted infections. Which of the following information should the nurse provide the client about using a contraceptive sponge? Select all that apply.

    a. Keep the sponge for more than 30 hours to prevent STIs

    b. Wet the sponge with water before inserting it

    c. Insert the sponge 24 hours before intercourse

    d. Leave the sponge in place for at least six hours following intercourse

    e. Replace sponge every two hours for the method to be effective

CHAPTER 5

Sexually Transmitted Infections

SECTION I: LEARNING OBJECTIVES

1. Define the key terms utilized in this chapter.

2. Construct the spread and control of sexually transmitted infections.

3. Identify risk factors and outline appropriate client education needed in common sexually transmitted infections.

4. Judge how contraceptives can play a role in the prevention of sexually transmitted infections.

5. Analyze the physiologic and psychological aspects of sexually transmitted infections.

6. Delineate the nursing management needed for women with sexually transmitted infections.

SECTION II: ASSESSING YOUR UNDERSTANDING

Activity A *Fill in the blanks.*

1. _____ is a common vaginal infection characterized by a heavy yellow, green, or gray frothy discharge.

2. The _____ stage of syphilis is characterized by diseases affecting the heart, eyes, brain, central nervous system, and/or skin.

3. _____ are a common cause of skin rash and pruritus throughout the world.

4. _____ is an intense pruritic dermatitis caused by a mite.

5. Vulvovaginal candidiasis, if not treated effectively during pregnancy, can cause the newborn to contract an oral infection known as _____ during the birth process.

6. _____ is a complex, curable bacterial infection caused by the spirochete *Treponema pallidum*.

7. Hepatitis B virus (HBV) can result in serious, permanent damage to the _____.

8. Cervicitis, acute urethral syndrome, salpingitis, PID, and infertility are conditions associated with _____ infection.

9. A person is said to be in the last stage of AIDS when the _____ T-cell count is less than or equal to 200.

10. Any woman suspected of having gonorrhea should be tested for _____ also, because co-infection (45%) is extremely common.

Activity B *Consider the following figures.*

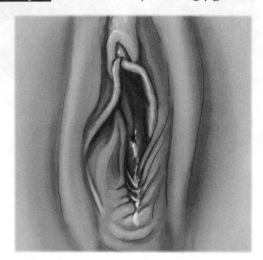

1. a. Identify this disease.

_____

_____

b. What is the consequence if this disease is untreated?

_____

_____

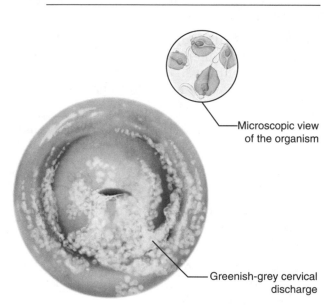

Microscopic view of the organism

Greenish-grey cervical discharge

2. a. Identify this disease.

_____

_____

b. What are the clinical manifestations of this disease?

_____

_____

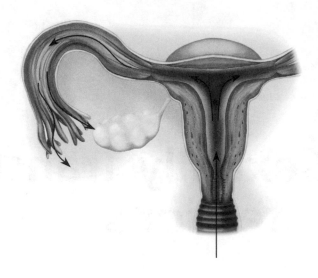

3. a. Identify the disease shown in the figure.

_____

_____

b. What are the causes of this disease?

_____

_____

Activity C *Match the sexually transmitted infections in Column A with their related descriptions in Column B.*

Column A

_____ **1.** Human immuno-deficiency virus (HIV)

_____ **2.** Vaginitis

_____ **3.** Hepatitis

_____ **4.** Gonorrhea

_____ **5.** Genital herpes

_____ **6.** Human papillomavirus (HPV)

Column B

a. Inflammation and infection of the vagina

b. Acute, systemic viral infection that can be transmitted sexually

c. Retrovirus causes breakdown in immune function, leading to acquired immunodeficiency syndrome (AIDS)

d. A recurrent, life-long viral infection

e. Cause of essentially all cases of cervical cancer

f. Very severe bacterial infection in the columnar epithelium of the endocervix

Activity D *Put the activities in correct sequence by writing the letters in the boxes provided below.*

1. Given below, in random order, are the manifestations of syphilis in its various stages. Arrange the stages in their correct order.

   a. Flu-like symptoms; rash on trunk, palms, and soles

   b. Life-threatening heart disease and neurologic disease that slowly destroys the heart, eyes, brain, central nervous system, and skin

   c. Painless ulcer at site of bacterial entry that disappears in 1 to 6 weeks

   d. No clinical manifestations even though serology is positive

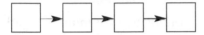

Activity E *Briefly answer the following.*

1. What are the predisposing factors for the occurrence of vulvovaginal candidiasis?

   _____

   _____

   _____

2. What are the symptoms of hepatitis A?

   _____

   _____

   _____

3. How is HIV transmitted?

   _____

   _____

   _____

4. What is acquired immunodeficiency syndrome (AIDS)?

   _____

   _____

   _____

5. What are the causes of vaginitis?

   _____

   _____

   _____

6. What are clinical manifestations of chlamydia?

   _____

   _____

   _____

SECTION III: APPLYING YOUR KNOWLEDGE

Activity F *Consider this scenario and answer the questions.*

1. A nurse is caring for a 22-year-old pregnant client who has been diagnosed with gonorrhea. The client seems to be very apprehensive about seeking treatment and wants to know if her newborn would be at risk for the infection.

   a. What information should the nurse provide the client regarding the transmission of the infection to the newborn?

   _____

   _____

   _____

   b. What factors should a nurse be aware of when caring for the client with gonorrhea or any other STI?

   _____

   _____

   _____

   c. Which groups of clients are at a higher risk for developing gonorrhea?

   _____

   _____

   _____

SECTION IV: PRACTICING FOR NCLEX

Activity G *Answer the following questions.*

1. A nurse is caring for a female client who has a history of recurring vulvovaginal candidiasis. Which of the following instructions should the nurse offer the client to prevent vulvo-vaginal candidiasis?

   a. Use superabsorbent tampons

   b. Douche the affected area regularly

   c. Wear white, 100% cotton underpants

   d. Increase intake of carbonated drinks

2. An HIV-positive client who is on antiretroviral therapy complains of anorexia, nausea, and vomiting. Which of the following suggestions should the nurse offer the client to cope with this condition?

   a. Use high-protein supplements

   b. Eat dry crackers after meals

   c. Limit number of meals to three a day

   d. Constantly drink fluids while eating

3. A client complaining of genital warts has been diagnosed with HPV. The genital warts have been treated, and they have disappeared. Which of the following should the nurse include in the teaching plan when educating the client about the condition?

   a. Applying steroid creams in affected area promotes comfort

   b. Even after warts are removed, HPV still remains

   c. All women above the age of 30 should get themselves vaccinated against HPV

   d. Use of latex condoms is associated with increased risk of cervical cancer

4. A female client is prescribed metronidazole for the treatment of trichomoniasis. Which of the following instructions should the nurse give the client undergoing treatment?

   a. Avoid extremes of temperature to the genital area

   b. Use condoms during sex

   c. Increase fluid intake

   d. Avoid alcohol

5. A nurse is required to assess a client complaining of unusual vaginal discharge for bacterial vaginosis. Which of the following is a classic manifestation of this condition that the nurse should assess for?

   a. Characteristic "stale fish" odor

   b. Heavy yellow discharge

   c. Dysfunctional uterine bleeding

   d. Erythema in the vulvovaginal area

6. A nurse needs to assess a female client for primary stage HSV infection. Which of the following symptoms related to this condition should the nurse assess for?

   a. Rashes on the face

   b. Yellow-green vaginal discharge

   c. Loss of hair or alopecia

   d. Genital vesicular lesions

7. A nurse working in a community health education program is assigned to educate community members about sexually transmitted infections. Which of the following nursing strategies should be adopted to prevent the spread of sexually transmitted infections in the community?

   a. Promote use of oral contraceptives

   b. Emphasize the importance of good body hygiene

   c. Discuss limiting the number of sex partners

   d. Emphasize not sharing personal items with others

8. A nurse who is conducting sessions on preventing the spread of sexually transmitted infections in a particular community discovers that there is a very high incidence of hepatitis B in the community. Which of the following measures should she take to ensure the prevention of hepatitis B?

   a. Ensure that the drinking water is disease-free

   b. Instruct people to get vaccinated for hepatitis B

   c. Educate about risks of injecting drugs

   d. Educate teenagers to delay onset of sexual activity

9. A nurse is caring for a client undergoing treatment for bacterial vaginosis. Which of the following instructions should the nurse give the client to prevent recurrence of bacterial vaginosis? Select all that apply.
   a. Practice monogamy
   b. Use oral contraceptives
   c. Avoid smoking
   d. Undergo colposcopy tests frequently

10. A pregnant client arrives at the community clinic complaining of fever blisters and cold sores on the lips, eyes, and face. The primary health care provider has diagnosed it as the primary episode of genital herpes simplex, for which antiviral therapy is recommended. Which of the following information should the nurse offer the client when educating her about managing the infection?
    a. Antiviral drug therapy cures the infection completely
    b. Kissing during the primary episode does not transmit the virus
    c. Safety of antiviral therapy during pregnancy has not been established
    d. Recurrent HSV infection episodes are longer and more severe

11. A 19-year-old female client has been diagnosed with pelvic inflammatory disease due to untreated gonorrhea. Which of the following instructions should the nurse offer when caring for the client? Select all that apply.
    a. Use an intrauterine device (IUD)
    b. Avoid douching vaginal area
    c. Complete the antibiotic therapy
    d. Increase fluid intake
    e. Limit the number of sex partners

12. A client complaining of genital ulcers has been diagnosed with syphilis. Which of the following nursing interventions should the nurse implement when caring for the client? Select all that apply.
    a. Have the client urinate in water if urination is painful
    b. Suggest the client apply ice packs to the genital area for comfort
    c. Instruct the client to wash her hands with soap and water after touching lesions

    d. Instruct the client to wear nonconstricting, comfortable clothes
    e. Instruct the client to abstain from sex during the latency period

13. A nurse is conducting an AIDS awareness program for women. Which of the following instructions should the nurse include in the teaching plan to empower women to develop control over their lives in a practical manner so that they can prevent becoming infected with HIV? Select the most appropriate responses.
    a. Give opportunities to practice negotiation techniques
    b. Encourage women to develop refusal skills
    c. Encourage women to use female condoms
    d. Support youth development activities to reduce sexual risk-taking
    e. Encourage women to lead a healthy lifestyle

14. A nurse is caring for an HIV-positive client who is on triple-combination HAART. Which of the following should the nurse include in the teaching plan when educating the client about the treatment? Select all that apply.
    a. Exposure of fetus to antiretroviral agents is completely safe
    b. Successful antiretroviral therapy may prevent AIDS
    c. Unpleasant side effects such as nausea and diarrhea are common
    d. Provide written materials describing diet, exercise, and medications
    e. Ensure that the client understands the dosing regimen and schedule

15. A nurse is caring for a female client who is undergoing treatment for genital warts due to HPV. Which of the following information should the nurse include when educating the client about the risk of cervical cancer? Select all that apply.
    a. Use of broad-spectrum antibiotics increases risk of cervical cancer
    b. Obtaining Pap smears regularly helps early detection of cervical cancer
    c. Abnormal vaginal discharge is a sign of cervical cancer
    d. Recurrence of genital warts increases risk of cervical cancer
    e. Use of latex condoms is associated with a lower rate of cervical cancer

16. A nurse is caring for a client who has just delivered a baby. Which of the following information should the nurse give the client regarding hepatitis B vaccination for the baby?

  a. Vaccine may not be safe for underweight or premature babies

  b. Vaccine consists of a series of three injections given within 6 months

  c. Vaccine is administered only after the infant is at least 6 months old

  d. Vaccine is required only if mother is identified as high-risk for hepatitis B

17. A pregnant client has been diagnosed with gonorrhea. Which of the following nursing interventions should be performed to prevent gonococcal ophthalmia neonatorum in the baby?

  a. Administer cephalosporins to mother during pregnancy

  b. Instill a prophylactic agent in the eyes of the newborn

  c. Perform a cesarean operation to prevent infection

  d. Administer an antiretroviral syrup to the newborn

18. A pregnant client is diagnosed with AIDS. Which of the following interventions should the nurse undertake to minimize the risk of transmission of AIDS to the infant?

  a. Ensure that the baby is delivered via cesarean

  b. Begin triple-combination HAART for the newborn

  c. Ensure that the baby is breastfed instead of being given formula

  d. Administer antiretroviral syrup to the infant within 12 hours after birth

CHAPTER 6

Disorders of the Breasts

SECTION I: LEARNING OBJECTIVES

1. Define the key terms utilized in this chapter.

2. Identify the incidence, risk factors, screening methods, and treatment modalities for benign breast conditions.

3. Outline preventive strategies for breast cancer through lifestyle changes and health screening.

4. Explain the incidence, risk factors, treatment modalities, and nursing considerations related to breast cancer.

5. Develop an educational plan to teach breast self-examination to a group of young women.

SECTION II: ASSESSING YOUR UNDERSTANDING

Activity A *Fill in the blanks.*

1. _____ is a useful adjunct to mammography that produces images of the breasts by sending sound waves through a conductive gel applied to the breasts.

2. _____, an alternative to radiation therapy, involves the use of a catheter to implant radioactive seeds into the breast after a tumor has been removed surgically.

3. Hormone therapy is used to block or counter the effect of the hormone _____ while treating breast cancer.

4. _____ is contraindicated for women whose active connective tissue conditions make them especially sensitive to the side effects of radiation.

5. _____ involves taking x-ray pictures of the breasts while they are compressed between two plastic plates.

6. _____, a type of therapy for breast cancer, leads to side effects such as hair loss, weight loss, and fatigue.

7. The removal of all breast tissue, the nipple, and the areola for breast cancer treatment is known as _____.

8. When diagnosing a woman with intraductal papilloma, a _____ card is used to evaluate nipple discharge for the presence of occult blood.

9. _____ is used as an adjunct therapy for breast cancer.

10. _____ are common benign solid breast tumors that occur in about 10% of all women and account for up to half of all breast biopsies.

Activity B *Consider the following figures.*

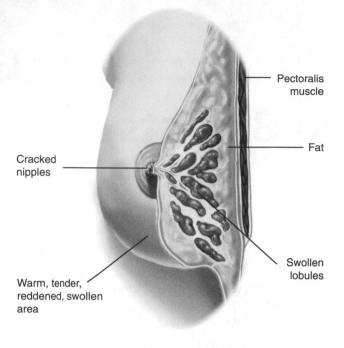

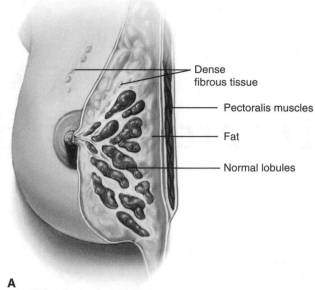

A

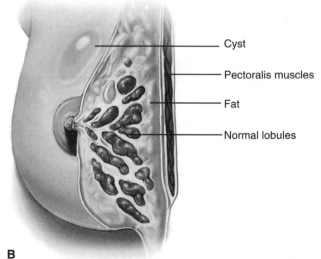

B

1. a. Identify the disease depicted in the figure above.

_____

_____

b. What are the clinical manifestations of this disease?

_____

_____

2. a. Identify the disease and the stage of disease depicted in each figure.

_____

_____

b. What are the clinical manifestations of the depicted disease stages?

_____

_____

Activity C *Match the benign breast disorders in Column A with their related descriptions in Column B.*

Column A

_____ **1.** Fibrocystic breast changes

_____ **2.** Fibroadenomas

_____ **3.** Intraductal papilloma

_____ **4.** Mammary duct ectasia

_____ **5.** Mastitis

Column B

a. An infection of the connective tissue in the breast, occurring primarily in lactating women

b. Dilation and inflammation of the ducts behind the nipple

c. Benign, wart-like growths found in the mammary ducts, usually near the nipple, caused by a proliferation and overgrowth of ductal epithelial tissue.

d. Firm, rubbery, well-circumscribed, freely mobile nodules that might or might not be tender when palpated

e. Lumpy, tender breasts; multiple, smooth, tiny "pebbles" or lumpy "oatmeal" under skin in later stages

Activity D *Briefly answer the following.*

1. What are benign breast disorders?

_____

_____

_____

2. What are the three aspects on which breast cancers are classified?

_____

_____

_____

3. What is breast-conserving surgery?

_____

_____

_____

4. What is adjunct therapy?

_____

_____

_____

5. What are the side effects of chemotherapy?

_____

_____

_____

6. Why is the status of the axillary lymph nodes important in the diagnosis of breast cancer?

_____

_____

_____

SECTION III: APPLYING YOUR KNOWLEDGE

Activity E *Consider this scenario and answer the questions.*

1. Mrs. Taylor, 54, presents to the women's health community clinic, where a nurse assesses her. She is very upset and crying. She tells the nurse that she found one large lump in her left breast and she knows that "it's cancer and I will die." When the nurse asks about her problem, she states that she does not routinely check her breasts and she hasn't had a mammogram for years because "they're too expensive." She also describes the intermittent pain she experiences in her breast.

a. What specific questions should the nurse include in her assessment of Mrs. Taylor?

_____

_____

_____

b. What education does Mrs. Taylor need regarding breast health?

_____

_____

_____

c. Explain what treatment modalities are available if Mrs. Taylor does have a malignancy.

_____

_____

_____

d. What community referrals are needed to meet Mrs. Taylor's future needs?

_____

_____

_____

SECTION IV: PRACTICING FOR NCLEX

Activity F *Answer the following questions.*

1. A client complains of lumpy, tender breasts, particularly during the week before menses. She complains of pain that often dissipates after the onset of menses. The nurse has to examine the client's breasts to confirm fibrocystic breast changes. Which of the following is the best time in the client's menstrual cycle to perform a breast examination?

   a. When the client is ovulating

   b. During the second phase of client's menstrual cycle

   c. A week after the client has completed her menses

   d. Immediately after the client's menses

2. A client arrives at the health care facility complaining of a lump that she felt during her breast self-examination. Upon diagnosis, the physician suspects fibroadenomas. Which of the following questions should the nurse ask when assessing the client?

   a. "Do you consume foods high in fat?"

   b. "Are you lactating?"

   c. "Are you taking oral contraceptives?"

   d. "Do you smoke regularly?"

3. A female client who has a two-month-old baby arrives at a health care facility complaining of flulike symptoms with fever and chills. When examining the breast, the nurse observes an increase in warmth, tenderness, and swelling with abraded nipples. The diagnosis indicates mastitis. Which of the following

instructions should the nurse provide the client to help her cope with the condition?

   a. Increase fluid intake

   b. Avoid breastfeeding for a month

   c. Avoid changing positions while nursing

   d. Apply cold compresses to the affected breast

4. Mammography is recommended for a client diagnosed with intraductal papilloma. Which of the following factors should the nurse ensure when preparing the client for a mammography?

   a. Client has not consumed fluids an hour prior to testing

   b. Client has not applied deodorant on the day of testing

   c. Client is just going to start her menses

   d. Client has taken an aspirin before the testing

5. A female client with a malignant tumor of the breast has to undergo chemotherapy for a period of 6 months. Which of the following side effects should the nurse monitor for when caring for this client?

   a. Vaginal discharge

   b. Headache

   c. Chills

   d. Constipation

6. A client diagnosed with fibroadenoma is worried about her chances of developing breast cancer. She also asks the nurse about various breast disorders and their risks. Which of the following benign breast disorders should the nurse mention as high risk for breast cancer?

   a. Fibrodenomas

   b. Mastitis

   c. Mammary duct ectasia

   d. Intraductal papilloma

7. It is recommended that a 48-year-old female client with breast cancer undergo a sentinel lymph node biopsy before lumpectomy. The client is anxious to know the reason for removing the sentinel lymph node. Which of the following information should the nurse offer the client?

   a. It will prevent lymphedema, which is a common side effect

   b. It will reveal the hormone-receptor status of the cancer

c. It will lessen the aggressiveness of the subsequent chemotherapy

d. It will allow the degree of HER-2/neu oncoprotein to be revealed

8. A client has undergone a mastectomy for breast cancer. Which of the following instructions should the nurse include in the post-surgery client-teaching plan?

a. Breathe rapidly for an hour

b. Elevate the affected arm on a pillow

c. Avoid moving the affected arm in any way

d. Restrict intake of medication

9. A 62-year-old female client arrives at a health care facility complaining of skin redness in the breast area, along with skin edema. The physician suspects inflammatory breast cancer. Which of the following is a symptom of inflammatory breast cancer that the nurse should assess for?

a. Palpable mobile cysts

b. Palpable papilloma

c. Increased warmth of the breast

d. Induced nipple discharge

10. A 41-year-old female client arrives at a health care setting complaining of dull nipple pain with a burning sensation, accompanied by pruritus around the nipple. The physician suspects mammary duct ectasia. Which of the following is a manifestation of mammary duct ectasia that the nurse should assess for?

a. Torturous tubular swellings in the upper half of breast

b. Increased warmth of the breasts, along with redness

c. Skin retractions on the breast when the skin is pulled

d. Green-colored nipple discharge with consistency of toothpaste

11. A 52-year-old female client with an ER+ breast cancer has to undergo hormonal therapy after her initial treatment. The client has to be administered selective estrogen receptor modulator (SERM). Which of the following side effects of SERM should the nurse monitor for when caring for the client?

a. Fever

b. Weight loss

c. Hot flashes

d. Chills

12. A nurse is assigned to educate a group of women on cancer awareness. Which of the following are the modifiable risk factors for breast cancer? Select all that apply.

a. Failing to breastfeed for up to a year after pregnancy

b. Early menarche or late menopause

c. Postmenopausal use of estrogen and progestins

d. Not having children until after age 30

e. Previous abnormal breast biopsy

13. A nurse is educating a client on the technique for performing breast self-examination. Which of the following instructions should the nurse include in the teaching plan with regard to the different degrees of pressure that need to be applied on the breast?

a. Light pressure midway into the tissue

b. Medium pressure around the areolar area

c. Medium pressure on the skin throughout

d. Hard pressure applied down to the ribs

14. A female client with metastatic breast disease is prescribed trastuzumab as part of her immunotherapy. Which of the following is the adverse effect of trastuzumab that a nurse should monitor for with the first infusion of the antibody?

a. Stroke

b. Hepatic failure

c. Myelosuppression

d. Dyspnea

15. A nurse is caring for a female client undergoing radiation therapy after her breast surgery. Which of the following is the side effect of radiation therapy that the client is likely to experience?

a. Anorexia

b. Infection

c. Fever

d. Nausea

16. A nurse is caring for a client who has just had her intraductal papilloma removed through a surgical procedure. What instructions should the nurse give this client as part of her care?

a. Apply warm compresses to the affected breast

b. Continue monthly breast self-examinations

c. Wear a supportive bra 24 hours a day

d. Refrain from consuming salt in diet

17. Lumpectomy is a treatment option for clients diagnosed with breast cancer with tumors smaller than 5 cm. For which of the following clients is lumpectomy contraindicated? Select all that apply.

    a. Client who has had an early menarche or late onset of menopause

    b. Client who has had previous radiation to the affected breast

    c. Client who has failed to breastfeed for up to a year after pregnancy

    d. Client whose connective tissue is reported to be sensitive to radiation

    e. Client whose surgery will not result in a clean margin of tissue

18. A 38-year-old female client has to undergo lymph node surgery in conjunction with mastectomy. The client is likely to experience lymphedema due to the surgery. Post-surgery, which of the following factors will make the client more susceptible to lymphedema? Select all that apply.

    a. Use of the affected arm for drawing blood or measuring blood pressure

    b. Engaging in activities like gardening without using gloves

    c. Not consuming foods that are rich in phytochemicals

    d. Not wearing a well-fitted compression sleeve

    e. Not consuming a diet high in fiber and protein

19. A 33-year-old female client complains of yellow nipple discharge and a pain in her breasts a week before menses that dissipates on the onset of menses. Diagnosis reveals that the client is experiencing fibrocystic breast changes. Which of the following instructions should the nurse offer the client to help alleviate the condition? Select all that apply.

    a. Increase fluid intake steadily

    b. Avoid caffeine

    c. Practice good hand-washing techniques

    d. Maintain a low-fat diet

    e. Take diuretics as recommended

20. A nurse is educating a 43-year-old female client about required lifestyle changes to help avoid breast cancer. Which of the following instructions regarding diet and food habits should the nurse include in the teaching plan? Select all that apply.

    a. Restrict intake of salted foods

    b. Limit intake of processed foods

    c. Consume seven or more portions of complex carbohydrates daily

    d. Increase liquid intake to 3 liters daily

    e. Consume at least five servings of proteins daily

CHAPTER 7

Benign Disorders of the Female Reproductive Tract

SECTION I: LEARNING OBJECTIVES

1. Define the key terms bolded throughout the chapter.

2. Identify the major pelvic relaxation disorders in terms of etiology, management, and nursing interventions.

3. Outline the nursing management needed for the most common benign reproductive disorders in women.

4. Relate the implications of urinary incontinence to future quality of life and to its pathology, clinical manifestations, and treatment options.

5. Compare the various benign growths to their symptomatology and course of management.

6. Explore the emotional impact on a woman diagnosed with polycystic ovarian syndrome and the nurse's role as a counselor, educator, and advocate.

SECTION II: ASSESSING YOUR UNDERSTANDING

Activity A *Fill in the blanks.*

1. _____ occurs when the posterior bladder wall protrudes downward through the anterior vaginal wall.

2. Uterine _____ occurs when the uterus descends through the pelvic floor and into the vaginal canal.

3. A _____ is a silicone or plastic device that is placed into the vagina to support the uterus, bladder, and rectum as a space-filling device.

4. _____ are small benign growths that may be associated with chronic inflammation, an abnormal local response to increased levels of estrogen, or local congestion of the cervical vasculature.

5. Uterine fibroids, or _____, are benign proliferations composed of smooth muscle and fibrous connective tissue in the uterus.

6. _____ exercises strengthen the pelvic-floor muscles to support the inner organs and prevent further prolapse.

7. Rectocele occurs when the _____ sags and pushes against or into the posterior vaginal wall.

8. Weakened pelvic floor musculature also prevents complete closure of the _____, resulting in urine leakage during moments of physical stress.

9. _____, or irregular, acyclic uterine bleeding, is the most frequent clinical manifestation of women with endometrial polyps.

10. _____ ultrasound is used to distinguish fluid-filled ovarian cysts from a solid malignancy.

Activity B *Consider the following figures.*

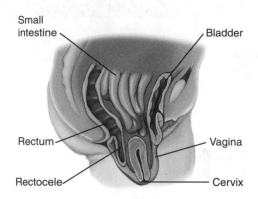

1. Identify the disorders, if any, shown in the figure.

_____

_____

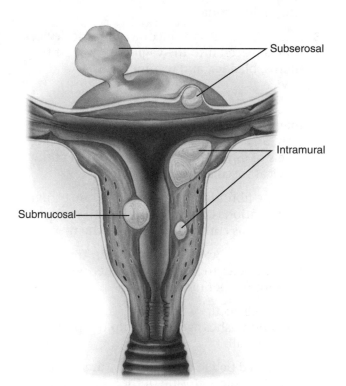

2. Identify the disorder in the figure.

_____

_____

Activity C *Match the benign disorders of the female reproductive tract in Column A with their correct definitions in Column B.*

Column A

____ **1.** Pelvic organ prolapse

____ **2.** Stress incontinence

____ **3.** Uterine fibroids

____ **4.** Polycystic ovarian syndrome

____ **5.** Urge incontinence

Column B

a. Abnormal descent or herniation of the pelvic organs from their original attachment sites or their normal positions in the pelvis

b. Benign tumors composed of muscular and fibrous tissue in the uterus

c. Presence of multiple inactive follicle cysts within the ovary that interfere with ovarian function

d. Precipitous loss of urine, preceded by a strong urge to void, with increased bladder pressure and detrusor contraction

e. Accidental leakage of urine that occurs with increased pressure on the bladder from coughing, sneezing, laughing, or physical exertion

Activity D *Briefly answer the following.*

1. What are the causes of pelvic organ prolapse?

_____

_____

_____

2. What are Kegel exercises?

_____

_____

_____

3. What are the causes of urinary incontinence?

_____

_____

_____

4. What is the Colpexin™ Sphere?

_____

_____

_____

5. What is uterine artery embolization (UAE)?

_____

_____

_____

6. What are Bartholin's cysts?

_____

_____

_____

SECTION III: APPLYING YOUR KNOWLEDGE

Activity E _Consider this scenario and answer the questions._

1. Mrs. Scott, age 57, comes in for her yearly gynecological examination and complains of "feeling like something is coming down in her vagina." She has chronic smoker's cough. Upon completion of a pelvic exam, uterine prolapse is diagnosed.

    a. What are the contributing factors to this disorder?

    _____

    _____

    _____

    b. What are the symptoms of uterine prolapse that may affect Mrs. Scott's daily activities?

    _____

    _____

    _____

    c. What are the nonsurgical and surgical interventions available to Mrs. Scott?

    _____

    _____

    _____

SECTION IV: PRACTICING FOR NCLEX

Activity F _Answer the following questions._

1. A 40-year-old client arrives at the community health center experiencing a strange dragging feeling in the vagina. At times, she feels as if there is a "lump" there as well. Which of the following conditions may be an indication of these symptoms?

    a. Urinary incontinence

    b. Endocervical polyps

    c. Pelvic organ prolapse

    d. Uterine fibroids

2. A nurse is caring for a client for whom estrogen replacement therapy has been recommended for pelvic organ prolapse. Which of the following is the most appropriate nursing intervention the nurse should implement before the start of the therapy?

    a. Discuss the effective dose of estrogen required to treat the client

    b. Evaluate the client to validate her risk for complications

    c. Discuss the dietary modifications following therapy

    d. Discuss the cost of estrogen replacement therapy

3. A nurse is caring for a female client with symptoms of early-stage pelvic organ prolapse. Which of the following instructions related to dietary and lifestyle modifications should the nurse provide to the client to help prevent pelvic relaxation and chronic problems later in life?

    a. Increase dietary fiber

    b. Avoid caffeine products

    c. Avoid excess intake of fluids

    d. Increase high-impact aerobics

4. Myomectomy is recommended to a client for removal of uterine fibroids. The client is concerned about the surgery and wants to know if there are any disadvantages associated with it. Which of the following is a disadvantage of myomectomy?

    a. Fertility is jeopardized

    b. Uterus is scarred and adhesions may form

    c. Uterine walls are weakened

    d. Fibroids may grow back

5. Kegel exercises are recommended for a client with pelvic organ prolapse. Of which of the following should the nurse inform the client about the exercises?

   a. They should be performed after food intake

   b. They alleviate mild prolapse symptoms

   c. They are not recommended after surgery

   d. They increase blood pressure

6. A nurse is assessing a 45-year-old client for uterine fibroids. Which of the following are the predisposing factors for uterine fibroids? Select all that apply.

   a. Age

   b. Nulliparity

   c. Smoking

   d. Obesity

   e. Hyperinsulinemia

7. A nurse is caring for a client who has been prescribed gonadotropin-releasing hormone (GnRH) medication for uterine fibroids. Which of the following is a side effect of GnRH medications that the nurse should monitor the client for?

   a. Increased vaginal discharge

   b. Vaginal dryness

   c. Urinary tract infections

   d. Vaginitis

8. A nurse is caring for a 32-year-old client for whom pessary usage is recommended for uterine prolapse. Which of the following instructions should the nurse include in the teaching plan for the client?

   a. Avoid jogging and jumping

   b. Wear a girdle or abdominal support

   c. Report any discomfort with urination

   d. Avoid lifting heavy objects

9. A nurse is caring for a 45-year-old client using a pessary to help decrease leakage of urine and support a prolapsed vagina. Which of the following is the most common recommendation a nurse should provide to the client regarding pessary care?

   a. Douche vaginal area with diluted vinegar or hydrogen peroxide

   b. Remove the pessary twice weekly, and clean it with soap and water

   c. Use estrogen cream to make the vaginal mucosa more resistant to erosion

   d. Remove the pessary before sleeping or intercourse

10. A client with abnormal uterine bleeding is diagnosed with small ovarian cysts. The nurse has to educate the client on the importance of routine check-ups. Which of the following is the most appropriate assessment for this client's condition?

    a. Monitor gonadotropin level every month

    b. Monitor blood sugar level every 15 days

    c. Schedule periodic Pap smears

    d. Schedule ultrasound every 3 to 6 months

11. A client with large uterine fibroids is scheduled to undergo a hysterectomy. Which of the following interventions should the nurse perform as a part of the preoperative care for the client?

    a. Teach turning, deep breathing, and coughing

    b. Instruct the client to reduce activity level

    c. Educate the client on the need for pelvic rest

    d. Instruct the client to avoid a high-fat diet

12. A 40-year-old client complains of low back pain after standing for a long time. The diagnosis reveals pelvic organ prolapse. The client has doubts regarding her eligibility for surgery. For which if the following clients is surgery for pelvic organ prolapse contraindicated? Select all that apply.

    a. Clients with low back pain and pelvic pressure

    b. Clients at high risk of recurrent prolapse after surgery

    c. Client who is morbidly obese before surgery

    d. Client who has severe pelvic organ prolapse

    e. Client who has chronic obstructive pulmonary disease

13. A nurse is caring for a female client with urinary incontinence. Which of the following instructions should the nurse include in the client's teaching plan to reduce the incidence or severity of incontinence? Select all that apply.

    a. Continue pelvic floor exercises

    b. Increase fiber in the diet

    c. Increase intake of orange juice

    d. Control blood glucose levels

    e. Wipe from back to front

14. A client has undergone an abdominal hysterectomy to remove uterine fibroids. Which of the followings interventions should a nurse perform as a part of the postoperative care for the client? Select all that apply.

   a. Administer analgesics promptly and use a PCA pump

   b. Avoid pillows and changing positions frequently

   c. Avoid intake of excess carbonated beverages in the diet

   d. Change linens and gown frequently to promote hygiene

   e. Administer antiemetics to control nausea and vomiting

15. A client with complaints of interference with normal voiding patterns and altered bowel habits is diagnosed with polycystic ovarian syndrome. Which of the following is the most appropriate instruction the nurse should provide to the client to help alleviate her condition?

   a. Adhere to follow-up care

   b. Increase intake of fiber-rich foods

   c. Increase fluid intake

   d. Perform Kegel exercises

CHAPTER 8

Cancers of the Female Reproductive Tract

SECTION I: LEARNING OBJECTIVES

1. Define the key terms addressed in the chapter.
2. Identify the major modifiable risk factors for reproductive tract cancers.
3. Examine the risk factors, screening methods, and treatment modalities for cancers of the reproductive tract.
4. Outline the nursing management needed for the most common malignant reproductive tract cancers in women.
5. Propose lifestyle changes and recommended health screenings needed to reduce risk or prevent reproductive tract cancers.
6. Investigate community resources available for the women undergoing surgery for a malignant reproductive condition.
7. Relate the psychological distress experienced by women diagnosed with cancer and the information needed to assist them to cope.

SECTION II: ASSESSING YOUR UNDERSTANDING

Activity A *Fill in the blanks.*

1. High-grade _____ can progress to invasive cervical cancer; the progression takes up to 2 years.

2. _____ is a microscopic examination of the lower genital tract with use of a magnifying instrument.

3. _____ is the use of liquid nitrogen to freeze abnormal cervical tissue.

4. _____ or uterine cancer is a malignant neoplastic growth of the uterine lining.

5. Pap smear results are classified by the _____ System.

6. _____ refers to the surgical removal of the uterus.

7. _____ is a biologic tumor marker associated with ovarian cancer.

8. The two major types of vulvar intraepithelial neoplasia (VIN) are classic (undifferentiated) and _____ (differentiated).

9. Ovarian cancer usually originates in the ovarian _____ .

10. _____ cell carcinomas that begin in the epithelial lining of the vagina tend to spread early by directly invading the bladder and rectal walls.

Activity B *Consider the following figures.*

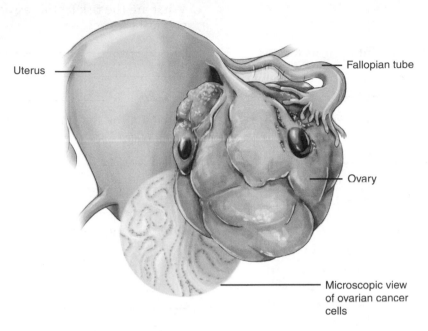

1. **a.** Identify the disorder shown in the image.

   _____

   _____

   b. What are the treatment options available for this disorder?

   _____

   _____

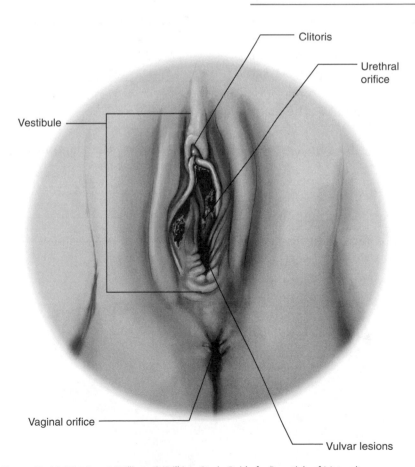

2. a. Identify the disorder shown in the image.

_____

_____

b. What are the treatment options for this disorder?

_____

_____

Activity C *Match the stages of endometrial cancer in Column A with the relevant organs affected during that stage in Column B.*

Column A

_____ **1.** Stage I

_____ **2.** Stage II

_____ **3.** Stage III

_____ **4.** Stage IV

Column B

a. Cervix

b. Muscle wall of the uterus

c. Bladder mucosa, with distant metastases to the lungs, liver, and bone

d. Bowel or vagina, with metastases to pelvic lymph nodes

Activity D *Put the items in correct sequence by writing the letters in the boxes provided below.*

Given below, in random order, are some of the steps performed by a nurse while assisting with the collection of a Pap smear. Choose the most likely sequence in which they would have occurred.

a. Provide support to the client as the practitioner obtains a sample

b. Drape the client with a sheet, leaving the perineal area exposed

c. Wash hands thoroughly

d. Transfer the specimen to a container or a slide

e. Position the client in stirrups or foot pedals so that her knees fall outward

f. Assemble the equipment, maintaining sterility of equipment

□ → □ → □ → □ → □ → □

Activity E *Briefly answer the following.*

1. What are the risk factors associated with cervical cancer?

_____

_____

_____

2. What are the treatment options for endometrial cancer?

_____

_____

_____

3. What are the risk factors for ovarian cancer?

_____

_____

_____

4. What is a transvaginal ultrasound used for?

_____

_____

_____

5. What are the nursing interventions when caring for clients with cancers of the female reproductive tract?

_____

_____

_____

6. What are the diagnostic options for endometrial cancer?

_____

_____

_____

SECTION III: APPLYING YOUR KNOWLEDGE

Activity F *Consider this scenario and answer the questions.*

1. Amy, age 60, has been diagnosed with ovarian cancer. Because this cancer develops slowly, remains silent, and is without symptoms until the cancer is far advanced, it is considered one of the worst gynecologic malignancies.

   a. What are the most common symptoms of ovarian cancer?

   _____

   _____

   _____

   b. There is still no adequate screening test to identify early cancer of the ovary. What suggestions should a nurse give a client to facilitate early detection of this type of cancer?

   _____

   _____

   _____

   c. State the nursing diagnoses related to malignancies of the reproductive tract.

   _____

   _____

   _____

   d. Explain the four stages of ovarian cancer.

   _____

   _____

   _____

SECTION IV: PRACTICING FOR NCLEX

Activity G *Answer the following questions.*

1. A nurse is educating a 25-year-old client with a family history of cervical cancer. Which of the following tests should the nurse inform the client about to detect cervical cancer at an early stage?

   a. Papanicolaou test

   b. Blood tests for mutations in the BRCA genes

   c. CA-125 blood test

   d. Transvaginal ultrasound

2. A client presents for her annual Pap test. She wants to know about the risk factors that are associated with cervical cancer. Which of the following should the nurse inform the client is a risk factor for cervical cancer?

   a. Early age at first intercourse

   b. Obesity (at least 50 pounds overweight)

   c. Hypertension

   d. Infertility

3. A client is waiting for the results of an endometrial biopsy for suspected endometrial cancer. She wants to know more about endometrial cancer and asks the nurse about the available treatment options. Which of the following treatment information should the nurse give the client?

   a. Surgery involves removal of the uterus only

   b. In advanced cancers, radiation and chemotherapy are used instead of surgery

   c. Surgery involves removal of the uterus, fallopian tubes, and ovaries; adjuvant therapy is used if relevant

   d. Follow-up care after the relevant treatment should last for at least 6 months after the treatment

4. A 65-year-old client presents at a local community health care center for a routine check-up. While obtaining her medical history, the nurse learns that the client had her menarche when she was 13 years old. She experienced menopause at 51. She is between 5 and 10 pounds underweight but is otherwise in good physical condition. The nurse should inform the client of which of the following factors that increase the client's risk of getting ovarian cancer?

   a. The client's age at menarche
   b. The client's present age
   c. The client's age at menopause
   d. The client's weight

5. A client presents at a community health care center for a routine check-up. The client wants to know about any tests that can effectively detect ovarian cancer early. About which of the following tests that can detect ovarian cancer should the nurse inform the client?

   a. Pap smears
   b. Serum CA-125
   c. Yearly bimanual pelvic examinations
   d. Regular x-rays of the pelvic area

6. A client presents for a routine check-up at a local health care center. One of the client's distant relatives died of ovarian cancer, and the client wants to know about measures that can reduce the risk of ovarian cancer. About which of the following measures to reduce the risk of ovarian cancer should the nurse inform the client?

   a. Provide genetic counseling and thorough assessment
   b. Instruct the client to avoid use of oral contraceptives
   c. Instruct the client to avoid breastfeeding
   d. Instruct the client to use perineal talc or hygiene sprays

7. A nurse is caring for a client who has been diagnosed with genital warts due to human papillomavirus (HPV). The nurse explains to the client that HPV increases the risk of vulvar cancer. Which of the following preventive measures to reduce the risk of vulvar cancer should the nurse explain to the client?

   a. Genital examination should be done only by the primary health care provider
   b. Genital examination should be done only by the client
   c. The client should avoid tight undergarments
   d. The client should use OTC drugs for self-medication of suspicious lesions
   e. The client should use oral contraceptives as opposed to barrier methods

8. When working in a local community health care center, a nurse is frequently asked about cervical cancer and ways to prevent it. Which of the following must the nurse advise regarding ways to reduce the risk of cervical cancer? Select all that apply.

   a. Encourage the use of an IUD for contraception
   b. Encourage cessation of smoking and drinking
   c. Encourage prevention of STIs to reduce risk factors
   d. Avoid stress and high blood pressure
   e. Counsel teenagers to avoid early sexual activity

9. The endometrial biopsy of a client reveals cancerous cells, and the primary health care provider has diagnosed it as endometrial cancer. Which of the following are responsibilities of the nurse as part of the treatment of the client? Select all that apply.

   a. Make sure the client understands all the available treatment options
   b. Inform the client that changes in sexuality are normal and need not be reported
   c. Inform the client about the possible advantages of a support group
   d. Offer the family explanations and emotional support throughout the treatment
   e. Inform the client that follow-up care is not required unless something unusual occurs

10. A nurse is conducting a session on education about cancers of the reproductive tract and is explaining the importance of visiting a health care professional if certain unusual symptoms appear. Which of the following should the nurse include in her list of symptoms that merit a visit to a health care professional for diagnosing cancers of the reproductive tract? Select all that apply.

    a. Irregular bowel movements

    b. Irregular vaginal bleeding

    c. Increase in urinary frequency

    d. Persistent low backache not related to standing

    e. Elevated or discolored vulvar lesions

11. A client has been referred for a colposcopy by the physician. The client wants to know more about the examination. Which of the following information regarding a colposcopy should the nurse give to the client?

    a. Client may feel pain in the vaginal area during the exam

    b. The test is conducted because of abnormal results in Pap smears

    c. Intercourse should be avoided for at least a week afterward

    d. Client may experience pain during urination for a week following the test

12. The results of a Pap smear test have been classified as ASC-H as per the 2001 Bethesda system. Which of the following is the correct interpretation of the result?

    a. Repeat the Pap smear in 4 to 6 months, or refer for a colposcopy

    b. Refer for a colposcopy without HPV testing

    c. Immediate colposcopy; follow-up is based on the results of findings

    d. No need for any further Pap smear screenings

13. Which of the following is the major initial symptom of endometrial cancer?

    a. Abnormal and painless vaginal bleeding

    b. Diabetes mellitus

    c. Liver disease

    d. Severe back pain

14. Which of the following risk factors are associated with vaginal cancer? Select all that apply.

    a. Advancing age

    b. HIV infection

    c. Persistent ovulation over time

    d. Smoking

    e. Hormone replacement therapy for more than 10 years

15. Which of the following risk factors has been linked to the development of vulvar cancer?

    a. Lichen sclerosus

    b. Previous pelvic radiation

    c. Exposure to diethylstilbestrol (DES) in utero

    d. Tamoxifen use

Violence and Abuse

SECTION I: LEARNING OBJECTIVES

1. Define the key terms bolded in the textbook chapter.

2. Evaluate the incidence of violence in women.

3. Outline the cycle of violence and appropriate interventions.

4. Critique the myths and facts about violence.

5. Analyze the dynamics of rape and sexual abuse.

6. Differentiate the resources available to women experiencing abuse.

7. Delineate the role of the nurse who cares for abused women.

SECTION II: ASSESSING YOUR UNDERSTANDING

Activity A *Fill in the blanks.*

1. A victim of _____ woman syndrome has experienced deliberate and repeated physical or sexual assault at the hands of an intimate partner.

2. _____ is any type of sexual exploitation between blood relatives or surrogate relatives before the victim reaches 18 years of age.

3. _____ rape is sexual activity between an adult and a person under the age of 18 and is considered to have occurred despite the willingness of the underage person.

4. _____, also known as roofies, forget pills, and the drop drug, is a common date rape drug.

5. Female genital mutilation, also known as female _____, refers to procedures involving the partial or total removal or other injury of the female genital organs.

6. _____ rape involves someone being forced to have sex by a person he or she knows.

7. Forcing objects into a woman's vagina against her will constitutes _____ abuse.

8. Increased emotional arousal, exaggerated startle response, and irritability are some of the symptoms of _____ during posttraumatic stress disorder (PTSD).

9. To assess for the presence of _____ reactions during posttraumatic stress disorder, the nurse should find out if the client feels numb emotionally or tries to avoid thinking of the trauma.

10. Victims of female genital mutilation are at an increased risk for _____ cysts.

Activity B *Match the four phases of rape recovery in Column A with the survivor's response in Column B.*

Column A

_____ **1.** Acute Phase (Disorganization)

_____ **2.** Outward Adjustment Phase (Denial)

_____ **3.** Reorganization

_____ **4.** Integration and Recovery

Column B

a. The survivor attempts to make life adjustments by moving or changing jobs and using emotional distancing to cope.

b. The survivor appears outwardly composed, refuses to discuss the assault, and denies need for counseling.

c. The survivor begins to feel safe, starts to trust others, and may become an advocate for other rape victims.

d. The survivor experiences shock, fear, disbelief, anger, shame, guilt, and feelings of being unclean

Activity C *Put the interventions in correct sequence by writing the letters in the boxes provided below.*

Given below are the interventions that a nurse performs when caring for a client who has been physically or sexually abused. Choose the order in which the interventions would have occurred.

a. Document and report findings

b. Screen for abuse during every health care visit

c. Isolate the client from her partner immediately

d. Ask direct and indirect questions about abuse

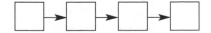

Activity D *Briefly answer the following.*

1. What is the cycle of violence?

_____

_____

_____

2. What is financial abuse?

_____

_____

_____

3. What are the potential nursing diagnoses related to violence against women?

_____

_____

_____

4. What is posttraumatic stress disorder (PTSD)? What are its symptoms?

_____

_____

_____

5. What signs should the nurse assess the client for, to find out if she is a victim of abuse?

_____

_____

_____

6. What are the effects of physical abuse on the pregnant woman?

_____

_____

_____

SECTION III: APPLYING YOUR KNOWLEDGE

Activity E *Consider this scenario and answer the questions.*

1. A visit to a health care agency is an ideal time for women to be assessed for violence. Suzanne, a married 24-year-old, presents to the Women's Center with complaints of pelvic pain, headaches, and sleep disruption. The triage nurse in the center recognizes that Suzanne became uncomfortable when discussing her marital relationship.

a. What are common symptoms of suspected physical abuse?

_____

_____

_____

b. Explain why Suzanne may not seek help when she is in an abusive relationship.

_____

_____

_____

c. What appropriate strategies should the nurse suggest that might help Suzanne to manage the situation?

_____

_____

_____

SECTION IV: PRACTICING FOR NCLEX

Activity F *Answer the following questions.*

1. A nurse is caring for a client who is being hospitalized for physical injuries. She later confides to the nurse that the injuries are a result of a physical assault by her partner when he was drunk. The client feels degraded and ashamed but realizes that her partner was under the influence of alcohol. How should the nurse respond to this client?

a. "Violent tendencies have gone on for generations; you need to accept it as part of life."

b. "Try to avoid provoking your partner in any way that might lead to abuse."

c. "Being drunk is not an excuse for physically assaulting an intimate partner."

d. "Violence occurs to only a small percentage of women who deserve it."

2. A client is receiving treatment for injuries sustained during a fight with her partner. The nurse observes that the partner visits her daily in the hospital and appears very solicitous and contrite. When questioned, she tries to convince the nurse that her partner is always very loving after a fight. Which of the following information should the nurse give to the client?

a. "No one deserves to be a victim of physical abuse."

b. "Your partner seems to be genuinely contrite."

c. "You should try not to upset your partner in the future."

d. "Don't worry; this is a normal part of any relationship."

3. A nurse is caring for a client who has been admitted with an ear infection. While discussing her partner with the nurse, the client says that her lover's behavior is "threatening" and "intimidating" at times, even though he has not physically harmed her. She wants to know what emotional abuse is. Which of the following should the nurse include as an example of emotional abuse while educating the client?

a. Being overly watchful of the client's every move

b. Throwing objects at the client

c. Destroying valued possessions or attacking pets

d. Forcing the client to have intercourse

4. A nurse is conducting an awareness session on sexual abuse, and she is explaining the psychological profile of an average abuser. Which of the following traits is displayed by abusers?

a. They have parents who are divorced

b. They exhibit antisocial behaviors

c. They belong to the low-income group

d. They are usually physically imposing

5. A nurse is working in a community hospital situated in an area with a history of grievous assaults on women, including rape. The nurse discovers that most rape victims come to the hospital but leave without seeking medical treatment. Which of the following interventions should the nurse perform to ensure that rape victims get legal and medical aid?

   a. Let them wait in waiting rooms to collect their thoughts before approaching them

   b. Treat them as any other client to make them feel more comfortable

   c. Focus on treating them rather than on collecting evidence

   d. Ensure that the appropriate law enforcement agencies are apprised of the incident

6. A client comes to a local community health care facility for a routine check-up. While talking to the nurse, the client happens to mention that every time she has a serious fight with her husband, he forces her to have intercourse with him. The client seems to be very disturbed when revealing this to the nurse. Which of the following is an appropriate response by the nurse?

   a. "Your husband is just trying to reconcile using intimacy."

   b. "It's okay in cases of fights where you're really at fault."

   c. "You need to be aware that you are being sexually abused."

   d. "Such behavior is considered normal in a married couple."

7. A 13-year-old immigrant from Asia is admitted to the health care facility with vaginal bleeding. An examination reveals that circumcision wounds have not healed. The client can understand English but cannot speak the language fluently. Hence, the service of an interpreter is employed. What are the points the nurse should keep in mind when interacting with this client?

   a. Convey important information in precise medical terms

   b. Allow the interpreter to question the client directly

   c. Use pictures and diagrams to assist the client's understanding

   d. Condemn the cultural practice and explain why it is wrong

8. A woman comes to a local community health care facility with her partner. She has a broken arm and bruises on the face that she claims were caused by a fall. However, the nature of the injuries causes the nurse to be convinced that this is a case of physical abuse. Which of the following interventions should the nurse perform?

   a. Ask the partner directly if he was responsible

   b. Attempt to interview the woman in private

   c. Tell the partner to leave the room immediately

   d. Question the client about the injury in front of the partner

9. A nurse is caring for a client who was raped at gunpoint. The client does not want any photos taken of her injuries. The client also does not want the police to be informed about the incident even though state laws require reporting life-threatening injuries. Which of the following interventions should the nurse perform to document and report the findings of the case?

   a. Use direct quotes and specific language when documenting

   b. Obtain photos to substantiate the client's case in a court of law

   c. Document only descriptions of medical interventions taken

   d. Respect the client's opinion and avoid informing the police

10. A nurse observes telltale signs of injuries from physical abuse on the face and neck of a female client. When questioned, the client tells the nurse that the injuries are the result of a physical attack by her partner and that she has developed palpitations thereafter. Which of the following should the nurse do to gain the trust of the client and enhance the nurse–client relationship?

    a. Offer referrals to the client so she can get help that will allow her to heal

    b. Tell the client to forget about the incident to avoid the trauma

    c. Inform the client that there is no connection between the violence and palpitations

    d. Confirm with the partner whether the client's story is true

11. A nurse is caring for a rape victim who has just arrived at the local health care facility. Which of the following interventions should the nurse perform to minimize risk of pregnancy in this client?

    a. Administer prescribed double dose of emergency contraceptive pills

    b. Wait for first signs of pregnancy before taking action

    c. Apply spermicidal cream or gel near the vaginal area

    d. Administer regular oral contraceptive pills

12. A nurse is caring for a pregnant client and discovers signs of bruises near her neck. On questioning, the nurse learns that the bruises were caused by her husband. The client tells the nurse that her husband had stopped abusing her some time ago, but this was the first time during the pregnancy that she was assaulted. She blames herself because she admits to not paying enough attention to her husband. Which of the following facts about abuse during pregnancy should the nurse tell the client to convince her that the abuse was not her fault? Select all that apply.

    a. Abuse is a result of concern for the unborn child when the mother doesn't fulfill her responsibilities toward the newborn

    b. Abuse is a result of resentment toward the interference of the growing fetus and change in the woman's shape

    c. Abuse is a result of the perception of the partner that the baby will be a competitor after he or she is born

    d. Abuse is a result of insecurity and jealousy of the pregnancy and the responsibilities it brings

    e. Most men exhibit violent reactions during pregnancy as a way of coping with the stress

13. A nurse is caring for a 16-year-old female immigrant. Which of the following questions must she ask the client to assess if she is a victim of human trafficking? Select all that apply.

    a. "Can you leave your job or situation if you wish?"

    b. "Can you come and go as you please?"

    c. "What is your education level?"

    d. "What do your parents and siblings do?"

    e. "Is there a lock on your door so you cannot get out?"

14. A nurse is working in a local community health care facility where she frequently encounters victims of abuse. Which of the following signs should the nurse assess for to find out if a client is a victim of abuse? Select all that apply.

    a. Client is affected by sexually transmitted infections frequently

    b. Client has mental health problems such as depression, anxiety, or substance abuse

    c. Client has injuries on the face, head, and neck

    d. Partner of the suspected victim seems relaxed and not overly worried

    e. The reported history of the injury is inconsistent with the actual presenting problem

15. A nurse is caring for a rape victim. Which of the following questions should the nurse ask the client to know the extent of physical symptoms of posttraumatic stress disorder (PTSD)? Select all that apply.

    a. "Are you having trouble sleeping?"

    b. "Have you felt irritable or experienced outbursts of anger?"

    c. "Do you have heart palpitations or sweating?"

    d. "Do you feel numb emotionally?"

    e. "Do upsetting thoughts and nightmares of the trauma bother you?"

CHAPTER 10

Fetal Development and Genetics

SECTION I: LEARNING OBJECTIVES

1. Describe the process of fertilization, implantation, and cell differentiation.

2. Explain the functions of the placenta, umbilical cord, and amniotic fluid.

3. Outline normal fetal development from conception through birth.

4. Compare the various inheritance patterns, including nontraditional patterns of inheritance.

5. Give examples of ethical and legal issues surrounding genetic testing.

6. Explain the role of the nurse in genetic counseling and genetic-related activities.

SECTION II: ASSESSING YOUR UNDERSTANDING

Activity A *Fill in the blanks.*

1. _____ is one of two or more alternative versions of a gene at a given position or locus on a chromosome that imparts the same characteristic of that gene.

2. Any change in gene structure or location leads to a _____, which may alter the type and amount of protein produced.

3. Human beings typically have 22 pairs of non-sex chromosomes or _____ and 1 pair of sex chromosomes.

4. The _____ originates from the ectoderm germ layer during the early stages of embryonic development; it is a thin protective membrane that contains the amniotic fluid.

5. _____ are long continuous strands of deoxyribonucleic acid (DNA) that carry genetic information.

6. The _____ reaches the uterine cavity about 72 hours after fertilization.

7. The pictorial analysis of the number, form, and size of an individual's chromosomes is termed _____.

8. _____ causes an increase in the number of haploid sets (23) of chromosomes in a cell.

9. A genetic disorder is a disease caused by an abnormality in an individual's genetic material or _____.

10. The genotype, together with environmental variation that influences the individual, determines the _____, or the observed, outward characteristics of an individual.

Activity B *Consider the following figures.*

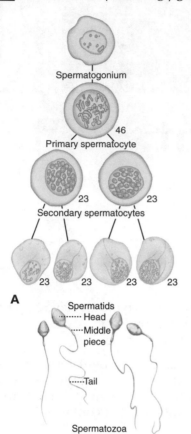

A

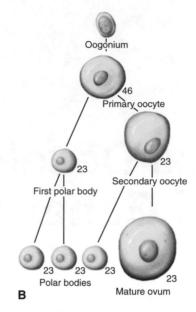

B

1. Identify the figure.

_____

_____

2. Identify the figure.

_____

_____

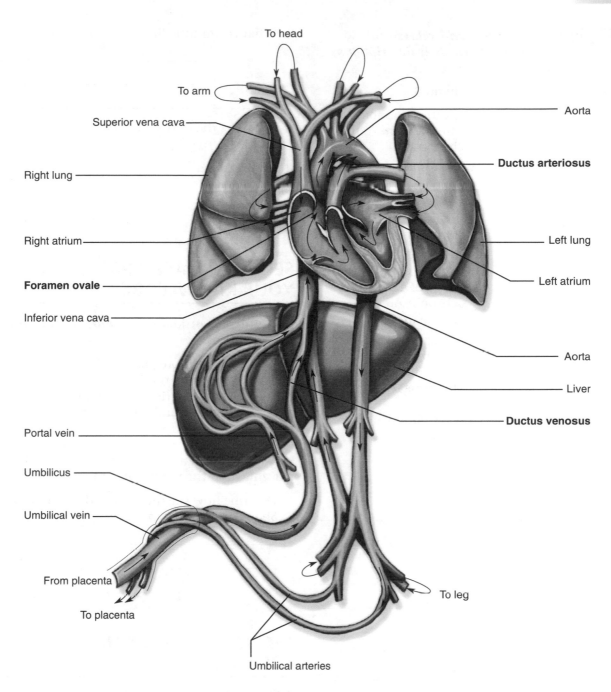

To head

To arm

Superior vena cava

Right lung

Right atrium

Foramen ovale

Inferior vena cava

Portal vein

Umbilicus

Umbilical vein

From placenta

To placenta

Umbilical arteries

Aorta

Ductus arteriosus

Left lung

Left atrium

Aorta

Liver

Ductus venosus

To leg

3. Identify the figure.

_____

_____

4. Explain the process in the figure.

_____

_____

Activity C *Match the terms related to genetics in Column A with their descriptions in Column B.*

Column A	Column B
____ **1.** Monosomies	**a.** Both alleles for a trait are the same in the individual
____ **2.** Trisomies	
____ **3.** Triploidy	**b.** Chromosomal abnormalities that do not show up in every cell
____ **4.** Mosaicism	
____ **5.** Homozygous	**c.** Three whole sets of chromosomes in a single cell
	d. There is only one copy of a particular chromosome instead of the usual pair
	e. There are three copies of a particular chromosome instead of the usual two

Activity D *Briefly answer the following.*

1. How does conception occur?

_____

_____

_____

2. What are the different stages of fetal development?

_____

_____

_____

3. What determines the sex of a zygote?

_____

_____

_____

4. What happens during differentiation of the zygote?

_____

_____

_____

5. What is amniotic fluid?

_____

_____

_____

6. What are the hormones produced by the placenta?

_____

_____

_____

SECTION III: APPLYING YOUR KNOWLEDGE

Activity E *Consider the scenario and answer the question.*

Shana is 16 weeks pregnant and comes into the prenatal clinic for a routine check-up. She tells the nurse she is worried because she feels the baby moving a lot and has concerns "it might get tangled in its cord." She wants to know if this could be true and, if so, why. Shana also wants to know about the functions of amniotic fluid, the placenta, and the umbilical cord.

1. Describe how the nurse should respond to Shana's questions and concern.

_____

_____

_____

SECTION IV: PRACTICING FOR NCLEX

Activity F *Answer the following questions.*

1. The nurse is counseling a couple who are concerned that the woman has achondroplasia in her family. The woman is not affected. Which of the following statements by the couple indicates the need for more teaching?

   a. "If the mother has the gene, then there is a 50% chance of passing it on."

   b. "If the father doesn't have the gene, then his son won't have achondroplasia."

c. "If the father has the gene, then there is a 50% chance of passing it on."

d. "Since neither one of us has the disorder, we won't pass it on."

2. A client has been informed that the result of the pregnancy test indicates that she is three weeks pregnant. Which of the following instructions should the nurse give to the client that is most appropriate given her condition?

a. Avoid exercising during pregnancy

b. Stay indoors and avoid going out for the duration of pregnancy

c. Instruct client to stop using drugs, alcohol, and tobacco

d. Wear comfortable clothes that are not tight or restrictive

3. A nurse is obtaining the genetic history of a pregnant client by questioning family members. Which of the following questions is most appropriate for the nurse to ask?

a. Were there any instances of premature birth in the family?

b. Is there a family history of drinking or drug abuse?

c. What was the cause and age of death for deceased family members?

d. Were there any instances of depression during pregnancy?

4. A nurse is caring for a 37-year-old pregnant client who is expecting twins, both boys. The client used to smoke but has stopped during pregnancy. A cousin of the client has Klinefelter syndrome, and the client wants to find out more about the disorder. Which of the following information will the nurse give to the client during genetic counseling?

a. There is a greater risk of Klinefelter syndrome due to the client's age

b. Klinefelter syndrome occurs only in girls and not boys

c. Having twins increases the risk of Klinefelter syndrome

d. The client's previous smoking habit will increase the risk of a genetic disorder

5. A 25-year-old client wants to know if her baby boy is at risk for Down syndrome, as one of her distant relatives was born with it. Which of the following will the nurse tell the client while counseling her about Down syndrome?

a. Instances of Down syndrome in the family increase the risk for the baby

b. Children with Down syndrome have 47 chromosomes instead of 46

c. Down syndrome occurs only in females, and there is no risk as the baby is male

d. Children with Down syndrome are intellectually normal

6. A nurse is questioning the family members of a pregnant client to obtain a genetic history. While asking questions, which of the following should the nurse keep in mind?

a. Inquire about the socioeconomic status of the family members

b. Avoid questions about race or ethnic background

c. Ask questions regarding physical characteristics of family members

d. Find out if couples are related to each other or have blood ties

7. A pregnant client and her husband have had a session with a genetic specialist. What is the role of the nurse after the client has seen a specialist?

a. Identify the best decision to be taken for the client

b. Refer the client to another specialist for a second opinion

c. Review what has been discussed with the specialist

d. Refer the client for further diagnostic and screening tests

8. A nurse is caring for a client who is pregnant with a female baby. The client and her husband are both in their early thirties. They are not directly related by blood. There has been an instance of Tay-Sachs disease occurring in the family. Which of the following information does the nurse need to give the client regarding Tay-Sachs disease?

a. Tay-Sachs disease affects both male and female babies

b. The age of the client increases the susceptibility of the baby to Tay-Sachs disease

c. There is no risk of Tay-Sachs disease because the parents are not related by blood

d. There is no risk of the baby developing Tay-Sachs disease because both parents are healthy

9. A pregnant client arrives at the community health center for a routine check-up. She informs the nurse that a relative on her mother's side has hemophilia, and she wants to know the chances of her child acquiring hemophilia. Which of the following characteristics of hemophilia should the nurse explain to the client to help her understand the odds of acquiring the disease? Select all that apply.

   a. Affected individuals will have affected parents

   b. Affected individuals are usually males

   c. Daughters of an affected male are unaffected and are not carriers

   d. Female carriers have a 50% chance of transmitting the disorder to their sons

   e. Females are affected by the condition if it is a dominant X-linked disorder

10. A nurse is providing genetic counseling to a pregnant client. Which of the following are the nursing responsibilities related to counseling the client? Select all that apply.

   a. Explaining basic concepts of probability and disorder susceptibility

   b. Ensuring complete informed consent to facilitate decisions about genetic testing

   c. Instructing the client on the appropriate decision to be taken

   d. Knowing basic genetic terminology and inheritance patterns

   e. Avoiding explaining ethical or legal issues and concentrating on genetic issues

Maternal Adaptation During Pregnancy

SECTION I: LEARNING OBJECTIVES

1. Define the key terms utilized in this chapter.

2. Differentiate between subjective (presumptive), objective (probable), and diagnostic (positive) signs of pregnancy.

3. Explain maternal physiologic changes that occur during pregnancy.

4. Summarize the nutritional needs of the pregnant woman and her fetus.

5. Identify the emotional and psychological changes that occur during pregnancy.

SECTION II: ASSESSING YOUR UNDERSTANDING

Activity A *Fill in the blanks.*

1. During the stress of pregnancy, _____, secreted by the adrenal glands, helps keep up the level of glucose in the plasma by breaking down noncarbohydrate sources.

2. _____, or having conflicting feelings at the same time, is an emotion expressed by most women upon learning they are pregnant.

3. _____, released by the posterior pituitary gland, is responsible for milk ejection during breastfeeding.

4. At birth, as soon as the _____ is expelled, and there is a drop in progesterone, lactogenesis can begin.

5. Palmar erythema, a well-delineated pinkish area on the palmar surface of the hands, is caused by elevated _____ levels.

6. The postural changes of pregnancy coupled with the loosening of the _____ joints may result in lower back pain.

7. Constipation, increased venous pressure, and pressure from the gravid uterus can lead to the formation of _____ during pregnancy.

8. During pregnancy, elevated _____ levels cause smooth-muscle relaxation, which results in delayed gastric emptying and decreased peristalsis.

9. _____ is the creamy, yellowish breast fluid that provides nourishment for the newborn during the first few days of life.

10. Most women experience an increase in a whitish vaginal discharge, called _____, during pregnancy.

Activity B *Consider the following figures.*

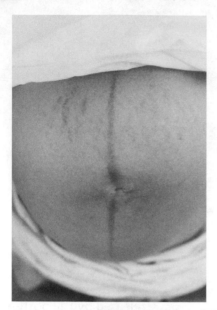

1. Identify the skin change shown in the image.

_____

_____

MyPyramid Plan for Moms

Food Group	1st Trimester	2nd and 3rd Trimesters	What counts as 1 cup or 1 ounce?	Remember to...
	Eat this amount from each group daily.*			
Fruits	2 cups	2 cups	1 cup fruit or juice, ½ cup dried fruit	*Focus on fruits*— Eat a variety of fruit.
Vegetables	2½ cups	3 cups	1 cup raw or cooked vegetables or juice, 2 cups raw leafy vegetables	*Vary your veggies*— Eat more dark green and orange vegetables and cooked dry beans.
Grains	6 ounces	8 ounces	1 slice bread; ½ cup cooked pasta, rice, cereal; 1 ounce ready-to-eat cereal	*Make half your grains whole*— Choose whole instead of refined grains.
Meat and Beans	5½ ounces	6½ ounces	1 ounce lean meat, poultry, fish; 1 egg; ¼ cup cooked dry beans; ½ ounce nuts; 1 tablespoon peanut butter	*Go lean with protein*—Choose low-fat or lean meats and poultry.
Milk	3 cups	3 cups	1 cup milk, 8 ounces yogurt, 1½ ounces cheese, 2 ounces processed cheese	*Get your calcium-rich foods*—Go low-fat or fat-free when you choose milk, yogurt, and cheese.

*These amounts are for an average pregnant woman. You may need more or less than the average. Check with your doctor to make sure you are gaining weight as you should.

2.

   a. What are the good food sources of folic acid?

_____

_____

   b. What foods does the FDA advise pregnant women and nursing mothers to avoid?

_____

_____

Activity C *Match the parts of the female reproductive tract in Column A with the physiologic changes that occur in them during pregnancy, in Column B.*

Column A

____ **1.** Uterus

____ **2.** Cervix

____ **3.** Vagina

____ **4.** Ovaries

____ **5.** Ureters

Column B

   a. Between weeks 6–8 of gestation, softens due to vasocongestion

   b. Elongate, widen, and curve above pelvic rim by tenth gestational week

   c. Connective tissue loosens and smooth muscle begins hypertrophy

   d. Produce more hormones until weeks 6–7 of gestation

   e. Weighs 2 lbs at full term

Activity D *Put the items in correct sequence by writing the letters in the boxes provided below.*

Given below, in random order, are the changes in the uterus as pregnancy progresses. Arrange the changes in sequence.

a. Uterus progressively ascends into the abdomen

b. Fundal height drops as fetus begins to descend and engage into the pelvis

c. Fundus reaches its highest level at the xiphoid process

d. Softening and compressibility of the lower uterine segment are noted

e. Fundus is at the level of the umbilicus and measures 20 cm

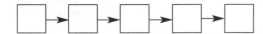

Activity E *Briefly answer the following.*

1. What are stretch marks?

_____

_____

_____

2. Why does hypertrophy of the heart occur in pregnant women?

_____

_____

_____

3. Why do iron requirements increase during pregnancy?

_____

_____

_____

4. What is pica?

_____

_____

_____

5. What is the role of oxytocin?

_____

_____

_____

6. Why do pregnant women develop varicose veins?

_____

_____

_____

SECTION III: APPLYING YOUR KNOWLEDGE

Activity F *Consider this scenario and answer the questions.*

1. A nurse working in a private doctor's office has been assigned to be the primary nurse for Maggie, 40, who is in her first trimester of pregnancy. Maggie states that she is very nervous about the pregnancy and is concerned because "she is not very excited." She adds that she is also worried about her baby, avoids travel, stays indoors because she feels nauseous most of the time, and has little interaction with the outside world. She asks the nurse if it is normal to feel this way.

a. Describe how the nurse should respond to the client about her lack of excitement.

_____

_____

_____

b. How should the nurse explain to the client how introversion, or focusing on oneself, may be common in early pregnancy?

_____

_____

_____

c. How should the nurse describe to the client how she may feel in the second trimester?

_____

_____

_____

d. How should the nurse reassure Maggie about her mood swings?

_____

_____

_____

SECTION IV: PRACTICING FOR NCLEX

Activity G *Answer the following questions.*

1. A 28-year-old client complains of skipping her menses and suspects she is pregnant. When assessing this client, which of the following would the nurse identify as a presumptive sign of pregnancy?

   a. Positive home pregnancy test

   b. Urinary frequency

   c. Abdominal enlargement

   d. Softening of the cervix

2. A pregnant client complains of an increase in a thick, whitish vaginal discharge. Which of the following information should a nurse provide to this client?

   a. Refrain from any sexual activity

   b. Consult physician for fungal infection

   c. Such discharge is normal during pregnancy

   d. Use local antifungal agents regularly

3. When teaching a client about hormones, which of the following should the nurse identify as responsible in developing the ductal system of the breasts in preparation for lactation during pregnancy?

   a. Estrogen

   b. Prolactin

   c. Progesterone

   d. Oxytocin

4. A 28-year-old client in her first trimester of pregnancy complains of conflicting feelings. She expresses feeling proud and excited about her pregnancy while at the same time feeling fearful and anxious of its implications. Which of the following maternal emotional responses is the client experiencing?

   a. Introversion

   b. Mood swings

   c. Acceptance

   d. Ambivalence

5. A pregnant client arrives at the maternity clinic complaining of constipation. Which of the following factors could be the cause of constipation during pregnancy? Select all that apply.

   a. Decreased activity level

   b. Increase in estrogen levels

   c. Use of iron supplements

   d. Reduced stomach acidity

   e. Intestinal displacement

6. A client in her 10th week of gestation arrives at the maternity clinic complaining of morning sickness. The nurse needs to inform the client about the body system adaptations during pregnancy. Which of the following factors corresponds to the morning sickness period during pregnancy?

   a. Reduced stomach acidity

   b. Elevation of hCG

c. Increase in RBC production

d. Increase in estrogen level

e. Elevation of hPL

7. A pregnant client in her first trimester of pregnancy complains of spontaneous, irregular, painless contractions. What does this indicate?

a. Preterm labor

b. Infection of the GI tract

c. Braxton Hicks contractions

d. Acid indigestion

8. A client in her 29th week of gestation complains of dizziness and clamminess when assuming a supine position. During the assessment, the nurse observes there is a marked decrease in the client's blood pressure. Which of the following interventions should the nurse implement to help alleviate this client's condition?

a. Keep the client's legs slightly elevated

b. Place the client in an orthopneic position

c. Keep the head of the client's bed slightly elevated

d. Place the client in the left lateral position

9. A client in her 20th week of gestation expresses concern about her five-year-old son, who is behaving strangely by not approaching her anymore. He does not seem to be taking the news of a new family member very well. Which of the following strategies can a nurse discuss with the mother to deal with the situation?

a. Provide constant reinforcement of love and care to the child

b. Avoid talking to the child about the new arrival

c. Pay less attention to the child to prepare him for the future

d. Consult a child psychologist about the situation

10. When caring for a newborn, the nurse observes that the neonate has developed white patches on the mucus membranes of the mouth. Which of the following conditions is the newborn most likely to be experiencing?

a. Rubella

b. Thrush

c. Cytomegalovirus infection

d. Toxoplasmosis

11. A client in her 39th week of gestation arrives at the maternity clinic stating that earlier in her pregnancy, she experienced shortness of breath. However, for the past few days, she's been able to breathe easily, but she has also begun to experience increased urinary frequency. A nurse is assigned to perform the physical examination of the client. Which of the following is the nurse most likely to observe?

a. Fundal height has dropped since the last recording

b. Fundal height is at its highest level at the xiphoid process

c. The fundus is at the level of the umbilicus and measures 20 cm

d. The lower uterine segment and cervix have softened

12. A client in her second trimester of pregnancy is anxious about the blotchy, brown pigmentation appearing on her forehead and cheeks. She also complains of increased pigmentation on her breasts and genitalia. When educating the client, which of the following would the nurse identify as the condition experienced by the client?

a. Linea nigra

b. Striae gravidarum

c. Facial melasma

d. Vascular spiders

13. A client in her 39th week of gestation complains of swelling in the legs after standing for long periods of time. The nurse recognizes that these factors increase the client's risk for which of the following conditions?

a. Hemorrhoids

b. Embolism

c. Venous thrombosis

d. Supine hypotension syndrome

14. A nurse is assigned to educate a pregnant client regarding the changes in the structures of the respiratory system taking place during pregnancy. Which of the following conditions are associated with such changes? Select all that apply.

a. Nasal and sinus stuffiness

b. Persistent cough

c. Nosebleed

d. Kussmaul's respirations

e. Thoracic rather than abdominal breathing

15. During a prenatal visit, a client in her second trimester of pregnancy verbalizes positive feelings about the pregnancy and conceptualizes the fetus. Which of the following is the most appropriate nursing intervention when the client expresses such feelings?

   a. Encourage the client to focus on herself, not on the fetus

   b. Inform the primary health care provider about the client's feeling

   c. Inform the client that it is too early to conceptualize the fetus

   d. Offer support and validation about the client's feelings

16. A client in her second trimester of pregnancy complains of discomfort during sexual activity. Which of the following instructions should a nurse provide?

   a. Perform frequent douching, and use lubricants

   b. Modify sexual positions to increase comfort

   c. Restrict contact to alternative, noncoital modes of sexual expression

   d. Perform stress-relieving and relaxing exercises

17. A nurse is educating a client about the various psychological feelings experienced by a woman and her partner during pregnancy. Which of the following is the feeling experienced by the expectant partner during the second trimester of pregnancy?

   a. Ambivalence along with extremes of emotions

   b. Confusion when dealing with the partner's mood swings

   c. Preparation for the new role as a parent and negotiating his or her role during labor

   d. Sympathetic response to the partner's pregnancy

CHAPTER 12

Nursing Management During Pregnancy

SECTION I: LEARNING OBJECTIVES

1. Define the key terms utilized in this chapter.

2. Identify the information typically collected at the initial prenatal visit.

3. Explain the assessments completed at follow-up prenatal visits.

4. Categorize the tests used to assess maternal and fetal well-being, including nursing management for each.

5. Outline appropriate nursing management to promote maternal self-care and minimize the common discomforts of pregnancy.

6. Design the key components of perinatal education.

SECTION II: ASSESSING YOUR UNDERSTANDING

Activity A *Fill in the blanks.*

1. A _____ is a laywoman trained to provide women and their families with encouragement, emotional and physical support, and information through late pregnancy, labor, and birth.

2. A _____ is a woman who has given birth once after a pregnancy of at least 20 weeks.

3. _____ height is the distance (in cm) measured with a tape measure from the top of the pubic bone to the top of the uterus while the client is lying on her back with her knees slightly flexed.

4. In a pregnant woman, darker pigmentation of the nipple and areola develops, along with enlargement of _____ glands in the breast.

5. Bluish coloration of the cervix and vaginal mucosa is known as _____ sign.

6. _____ is the craving for nonfood substances such as clay, cornstarch, laundry detergent, baking soda, soap, paint chips, dirt, ice, or wax.

7. _____ involves a transabdominal perforation of the amniotic sac to obtain a sample of amniotic fluid for analysis.

8. Alpha-fetoprotein (AFP) is a substance produced by the fetal _____ between weeks 13 and 20 of gestation.

9. The basis for the _____ test is that the normal fetus produces characteristic fetal heart rate patterns in response to fetal movements.

10. _____ are varicosities of the rectum which occur as a result of progesterone-induced vasodilation and from pressure of the enlarged uterus on the lower intestine and rectum.

Activity B *Consider the following figures.*

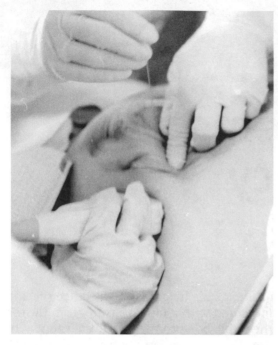

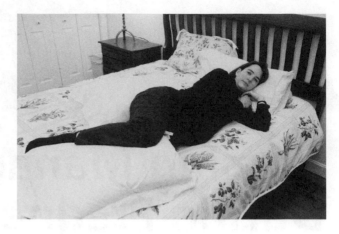

2. a. Identify the figure.

_____

_____

b. Why is this important for the client?

_____

_____

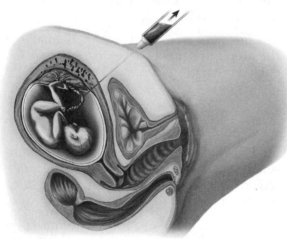

1. a. Identify the technique shown in the figure.

_____

_____

b. What is this technique used for?

_____

_____

Activity C *Match the different types of assessment tests conducted to determine fetal well-being, in Column A, with their uses in Column B.*

Column A

_____ **1.** 1. Ultrasonography

_____ **2.** Doppler flow studies

_____ **3.** Nuchal translucency screening (ultrasound)

_____ **4.** Percutaneous umbilical blood sampling (PUBS)

_____ **5.** Contraction stress test (CST)

Column B

a. Allows for earlier detection and diagnosis of some fetal chromosomes and structural abnormalities

b. Permits the collection of a blood specimen directly from the fetal circulation for rapid chromosomal analysis.

c. Determines the fetal heart rate response under stress, such as during contractions.

d. Acts as a guide for the need for invasive intrauterine tests and used to monitor fetal growth and placental location.

e. Help to identify abnormalities in diastolic flow within the umbilical vessels

Activity D *Put the steps in correct sequence by writing the letters in the boxes provided below.*

Given below, in random order, are steps that should be followed by the client who has nosebleeds. Rearrange in the correct sequence.

a. Pinch her nostrils with her thumb and forefinger for 10 to 15 minutes

b. Loosen the clothing around her neck

c. Apply an ice pack to the bridge of her nose

d. Sit with her head tilted forward

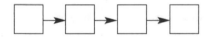

Activity E *Briefly answer the following.*

1. What are the key areas which the nurse should include in preconception care?

_____

_____

_____

2. What is the role of a nurse in preconception care to ensure a positive impact on the pregnancy?

_____

_____

_____

3. What are the assessments the nurse should make during a client's initial prenatal visit?

_____

_____

_____

4. What are the roles of a nurse with regard to providing counseling and education to the client at a prenatal visit?

_____

_____

_____

5. What assessments should a nurse perform when conducting a chest examination for a pregnant client on her first prenatal visit?

_____

_____

_____

6. What assessments should the nurse perform during follow-up visits?

_____

_____

_____

SECTION III: APPLYING YOUR KNOWLEDGE

Activity F *Consider this scenario and answer the questions.*

1. A pregnant client and her husband are preparing for the birth of their first baby. The couple wants to ensure that they are well prepared for the baby's birth and homecoming and seek guidance from the nurse. The pregnant client also wants to know the importance of breastfeeding and wants to prepare for it.

a. What are the items in the checklist used by the nurse to ensure that the client is well prepared for the newborn's birth and homecoming?

_____

_____

_____

b. What interventions should the nurse perform in preparing the client for breastfeeding?

_____

_____

_____

c. What advantages of breastfeeding should the nurse educate the pregnant client about?

_____

_____

_____

SECTION IV: PRACTICING FOR NCLEX

Activity G *Answer the following questions.*

1. A 28-year-old client who has just conceived arrives at a health care facility for her first prenatal visit to undergo a physical examination. Which of the following interventions should the nurse perform to prepare the client for the physical examination?

   a. Ensure that the client is lying down
   b. Ensure that the client's family is present
   c. Instruct the client to empty her bladder
   d. Instruct the client to keep taking deep breaths

2. A client in her third month of pregnancy arrives at the health care facility for a regular follow-up visit. The client complains of discomfort due to increased urinary frequency. Which of the following instructions should the nurse offer the client to reduce the client's discomfort?

   a. Avoid consumption of caffeinated drinks
   b. Drink fluids with meals rather than between meals
   c. Avoid an empty stomach at all times
   d. Munch on dry crackers and toast in the early morning

3. A pregnant client has come to a health care provider for her first prenatal visit. The nurse needs to document useful information about the past health history. What is the goal of the nurse in the history-taking process? Select all that apply.

   a. To prepare a plan of care that suits the client's lifestyle
   b. To develop a trusting relationship with the client
   c. To prepare a plan of care for the pregnancy

   d. To assess the client's partner's sexual health
   e. To urge the client to achieve an optimal body weight

4. A pregnant client has come to a health care facility for a physical examination. Which of the following assessments should a nurse perform when doing a physical examination of the head and neck? Select all that apply.

   a. Assess for previous injuries and sequelae
   b. Check the eye movements
   c. Check for levels of estrogen
   d. Evaluate for limitations in range of motion
   e. Palpate the thyroid gland for enlargement

5. A pregnant client in her 12th week of gestation has come to a health care center for a physical examination of her abdomen. Where should the nurse palpate for the fundus in this client?

   a. At the umbilicus
   b. Below the ensiform cartilage
   c. Midway between the symphysis and umbilicus
   d. At the symphysis pubis

6. A pregnant client has come to a clinic for a pelvic examination. What assessments should a nurse perform when examining external genitalia?

   a. Ensure that the cervix is smooth, long, thick, and closed
   b. Assess for bluish coloration of cervix and vaginal mucosa
   c. Assess for any infection due to hematomas, varicosities, and inflammation
   d. Assess for hemorrhoids, masses, prolapse, and lesions

7. Which of the following nursing interventions should the nurse perform when assessing fetal well-being through abdominal ultrasonography in a client?

   a. Inform the client that she may feel hot initially
   b. Instruct the client to refrain from emptying her bladder
   c. Instruct the client to report the occurrence of fever
   d. Obtain and record vital signs of the client

8. A pregnant client wishes to know if sexual intercourse would be safe during her pregnancy. Which of the following should the nurse confirm before educating the client regarding sexual behavior during pregnancy?

   a. Client does not have an incompetent cervix

   b. Client does not have anxieties and worries

   c. Client does not have anemia

   d. Client does not experience facial and hand edema

9. A client in her second trimester arrives at a health care facility for a follow-up visit. During the exam, the client complains of constipation. Which of the following instructions should the nurse offer to help alleviate constipation?

   a. Ensure adequate hydration and bulk in the diet

   b. Avoid spicy or greasy foods in meals

   c. Practice Kegel exercises

   d. Avoid lying down for two hours after meals

10. A client in the third trimester of pregnancy has to travel a long distance by car. The client is anxious about the effect the travel may have on her pregnancy. Which of the following instructions should the nurse provide to promote easy and safe travel for the client?

    a. Activate the air bag in the car

    b. Use a lap belt that crosses over the uterus

    c. Apply a padded shoulder strap properly

    d. Always wear a three-point seat belt

11. A pregnant client's last menstrual period was March 10. Using Nagele's rule, the nurse knows that which of the following dates should be the client's estimated date of birth (EDB)?

    a. January 7

    b. December 17

    c. February 21

    d. January 30

12. A nurse who has been caring for a pregnant client understands that the client has pica and has been regularly consuming soil. Which of the following conditions should the nurse monitor for in the client as a manifestation of consuming soil?

    a. Iron-deficiency anemia

    b. Constipation

    c. Tooth fracture

    d. Inefficient protein metabolism

13. A client who has just conceived arrives at a health care facility wanting to know of any changes in her eating habits that she should make during her pregnancy. The client informs the nurse that she is a vegetarian. The nurse knows that she has to monitor the client for which of the following risks arising from her vegetarian diet? Select all that apply.

    a. Risk of epistaxis

    b. Iron-deficiency anemia

    c. Decreased mineral absorption

    d. Increased risk of constipation

    e. Low gestational weight gain

14. A nurse is caring for a pregnant client in her second trimester of pregnancy. The nurse educates the client to look for which of the following danger signs of pregnancy needing immediate attention by the physician.

    a. Vaginal bleeding

    b. Painful urination

    c. Severe, persistent vomiting

    d. Lower abdominal and shoulder pain

15. A client in her third trimester of pregnancy wishes to use the method of feeding formula to her infant. Which of the following instructions should the nurse provide to assist the client in feeding her baby?

    a. Mix one scoop of powder with an ounce of water

    b. Feed the infant every 8 hours

    c. Serve the formula at room temperature

    d. Refrigerate any leftover formula

16. A nurse caring for a client in labor has asked her to perform Lamaze breathing techniques to avoid pain. Which of the following should the nurse keep in mind to promote effective Lamaze method breathing?

    a. Ensure deep abdominopelvic breathing

    b. Ensure abdominal breathing during contractions

    c. Ensure client's concentration on pleasurable sensations

    d. Remain quiet during client's period of imagery

17. A nurse is caring for a client in her second trimester of pregnancy. During a regular follow-up visit, the client complains of varicosities of the legs. Which of the following instructions should the nurse provide to help the client alleviate varicosities of the legs?

a. Avoid sitting in one position for long

b. Refrain from crossing legs when sitting for long periods

c. Apply heating pads on the extremities

d. Refrain from wearing any kind of stockings

18. A nurse is assigned to care for a pregnant client as she undergoes a nonstress test. Given below are the steps involved in conducting the nonstress test. Arrange the steps in correct order.

a. Client is handed an event marker

b. Client consumes a meal

c. External electronic fetal monitoring device applied

d. Fetal monitor strip marked for fetal movement

e. Client placed in left lateral recumbent position

CHAPTER 13

Labor and Birth Process

SECTION I: LEARNING OBJECTIVES

1. Outline premonitory signs of labor.

2. Compare and contrast true versus false labor.

3. Categorize the critical factors affecting labor and birth.

4. Analyze the cardinal movements of labor.

5. Identify the maternal and fetal responses to labor and birth.

6. Classify the stages of labor and the critical events in each stage.

7. Explain the normal physiologic/psychological changes occurring during all four stages of labor.

8. Formulate the concept of pain as it relates to the woman in labor.

SECTION II: ASSESSING YOUR UNDERSTANDING

Activity A *Fill in the blanks.*

1. Vaginal birth is most favorable with a _____ type of pelvis because the inlet is round and the outlet is roomy.

2. The thinning out process of the cervix during labor is termed _____.

3. The _____ suture is located between the parietal bones and divides the skull into the right and left halves.

4. _____ station is designated when the presenting part is at the level of the maternal ischial spines.

5. _____ occurs when the fetal presenting part begins to descend into the maternal pelvis.

6. An increase in prostaglandins leads to myometrial _____ and to a reduction in cervical resistance.

7. Oxytocin also aids in stimulating prostaglandin synthesis through receptors in the _____.

8. The birth _____ is the route through which the fetus must travel to be birthed vaginally.

9. A sudden increase in energy on the part of the expectant woman 24 to 48 hours before the onset of labor is sometimes referred to as _____.

10. The elongated shape of the fetal skull at birth as a result of overlapping of the cranial bones is known as _____.

Activity B *Consider the following figures.*

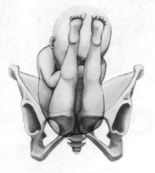

1. a. Identify the figure.

_____

_____

b. In which clients are such cases observed?

_____

_____

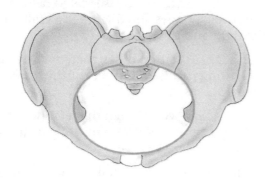

2. a. Identify the figure.

_____

_____

b. What are the possible complications associated with this condition?

_____

_____

Activity C *Match the cardinal movements of labor in Column A with the corresponding fetal movements observed in Column B.*

Column A

Column B

____ **1.** Engagement

____ **2.** Descent

____ **3.** Flexion

a. Occurs when the greatest transverse diameter of the head in vertex passes through the pelvic inlet

____ **4.** Extension

____ **5.** External rotation

b. Downward movement of the fetal head until it is within the pelvic inlet

c. Allows the shoulders to rotate internally to fit the maternal pelvis

d. The head emerges through extension under the symphysis pubis, along with the shoulders

e. Occurs as the vertex meets resistance from the cervix, walls of the pelvis, or the pelvic floor

Activity D *Put the items in correct sequence by writing the letters in the boxes provided below.*

Given below, in random order, are the phases of labor. Arrange them in the order of their occurrence.

a. Latent phase

b. Active phase

c. Transition phase

d. Pelvic phase

e. Perineal phase

f. Placental separation

g. Placental expulsion

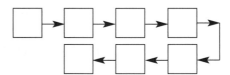

Activity E *Briefly answer the following.*

1. What are the reasons that cause women to adopt back-lying positions during labor?

_____

_____

_____

2. Why should the nurse encourage the pregnant client experiencing contractions to adopt the upright or lateral position?

_____

_____

_____

3. What are the maternal physiologic responses that occur as a woman progresses through childbirth?

_____

_____

_____

4. What are the factors influencing the ability of a woman to cope with labor stress?

_____

_____

_____

5. What are the signs of separation that indicate the placenta is ready to deliver?

_____

_____

_____

6. What are the factors that ensure a positive birth experience for the pregnant client?

_____

_____

_____

SECTION III: APPLYING YOUR KNOWLEDGE

Activity F *Consider this scenario and answer the questions.*

1. Becca is a primigravida at 36 weeks' gestation. During her prenatal visit, she asks the nurse the following questions about labor. Describe how the nurse should respond.

a. "How will I know I am in labor?"

_____

_____

b. "When should I come to the hospital?"

_____

_____

_____

c. "My sister just had a baby and she told me that the nurse midwife encouraged her to change positions and to walk to help her labor; will this help me in labor?"

_____

_____

_____

d. "How do we determine that it's time to push?"

_____

_____

_____

SECTION IV: PRACTICING FOR NCLEX

Activity G *Answer the following questions.*

1. A client in her third trimester of pregnancy arrives at a health care facility complaining of cramping and low back pain. Physical examination conducted by the nurse indicates that the client has edema of the lower extremities, along with an increase in vaginal discharge. The nurse knows that the client is experiencing which of the following conditions?

a. Nesting

b. Lightening

c. Braxton Hicks contractions

d. Bloody show

2. A pregnant client who is toward the end of her third trimester presents at a health care facility for a follow-up visit. Assessment of the client reveals that she has increased prostaglandin levels. Which of the following factors should the nurse assess for in the client? Select all that apply.

a. Reduction in cervical resistance

b. Myometrial contractions

c. Boggy appearance of the uterus

d. Softening and thinning of the cervix

e. Hypotonic character of the bladder

3. A client experiencing contractions presents at a health care facility. Assessment conducted by the nurse reveals that the client has been experiencing Braxton Hicks contractions. The nurse has to educate the client on the usefulness of Braxton Hicks contractions. Which of the following is the role of Braxton Hicks contractions in aiding labor?

   a. Helps in softening and ripening the cervix

   b. Increases the release of prostaglandins

   c. Increases oxytocin sensitivity

   d. Makes maternal breathing easier

4. A pregnant client wants to know why the labor of a first-time-pregnant woman lasts longer than that of a woman who has already delivered once and is pregnant a second time. What explanation should the nurse offer the client?

   a. Braxton Hicks contractions are not strong enough during first pregnancy

   b. Contractions are stronger during the first pregnancy than the second

   c. The cervix takes around 12 to 16 hours to dilate during first pregnancy

   d. Spontaneous rupture of membranes occurs during first pregnancy

5. A pregnant client is admitted to a maternity clinic for childbirth. The client wishes to adopt the kneeling position during labor. The nurse knows that which of the following is the advantage of adopting a kneeling position during labor?

   a. It helps the woman in labor to save energy

   b. It facilitates vaginal examinations

   c. It facilitates external belt adjustment

   d. It helps to rotate fetus in a posterior position

6. A nurse is caring for a pregnant client who is in labor. Which of the following maternal physiologic responses should the nurse monitor for in the client as the client progresses through childbirth? Select all that apply.

   a. Increase in heart rate

   b. Increase in blood pressure

   c. Increase in respiratory rate

   d. Slight decrease in body temperature

   e. Increase in gastric emptying and pH

7. A nurse is caring for a client in labor who is delivering. Which of the following fetal responses should the nurse monitor for in the client's baby?

   a. Decrease in arterial carbon dioxide pressure

   b. Increase in fetal breathing movements

   c. Increase in fetal oxygen pressure

   d. Decrease in circulation and perfusion to the fetus

8. A client in the third stage of labor has experienced placental separation and expulsion. Why is it necessary for a nurse to massage the woman's uterus briefly until it is firm?

   a. To reduce boggy nature of the uterus

   b. To remove pieces left attached to uterine wall

   c. To constrict the uterine blood vessels

   d. To lessen the chances of conducting an episiotomy

9. A nurse is caring for a pregnant client in labor in a health care facility. The nurse knows that which of the following marks the termination of the first stage of labor in the client?

   a. Diffuse abdominal cramping

   b. Rupturing of fetal membranes

   c. Start of regular contractions

   d. Dilation of cervix diameter to 10 cm

10. A nurse is caring for a client who is in the first stage of labor. The client is experiencing extreme pain due to the labor. The nurse understands that which of the following is causing the extreme pain in the client? Select all that apply.

    a. Lower uterine segment distention

    b. Fetus moving along the birth canal

    c. Stretching and tearing of structures

    d. Spontaneous placental expulsion

    e. Dilation of the cervix

11. A pregnant client in labor has to undergo a sonogram to confirm the fetal position of a shoulder presentation. The nurse has to assess for which of the following conditions associated with shoulder presentation during a vaginal birth?

    a. Uterine abnormalities

    b. Fetal anomalies

    c. Congenital anomalies

    d. Prematurity

12. A nurse is assigned the task of educating a pregnant client about childbirth. Which of the following nursing interventions should the nurse perform as a part of prenatal education for the client to ensure a positive childbirth experience? Select all that apply.

    a. Provide the client clear information on procedures involved

    b. Encourage the client to have a sense of mastery and self-control

    c. Encourage the client to have a positive reaction to pregnancy

    d. Instruct the client to spend some time alone each day

    e. Instruct the client to begin changing the home environment

13. A pregnant client is admitted to a maternity clinic for childbirth. What should the assigned nurse observe to conclude that the client's fetus is in the transverse lie position?

    a. Long axis of fetus is at 60 degrees to that of client

    b. Long axis of fetus is parallel to that of client

    c. Long axis of fetus is perpendicular to that of client

    d. Long axis of fetus is at 45 degrees to that of client

14. A pregnant client is admitted to a maternity clinic after experiencing contractions. The assigned nurse observes that the client experiences pauses between contractions. The nurse knows that which of the following marks the importance of the pauses between contractions during labor?

    a. Effacement and dilation of the cervix

    b. Shortening of the upper uterine segment

    c. Reduction in length of the cervical canal

    d. Restoration of blood flow to uterus and placenta

15. A pregnant client is admitted to a maternity clinic for delivery. Which of the following conditions should the nurse observe in the client during a vaginal birth to identify shoulder presentation?

    a. Multiparity

    b. Uterine abnormalities

    c. Multiple gestation

    d. Congenital anomalies

16. A nurse is caring for a pregnant client during labor. Which of the following methods should the nurse use to provide comfort to the pregnant client? Select all that apply.

    a. Hand holding

    b. Chewing gum

    c. Massaging

    d. Acupressure

    e. Prescribed pain killers

CHAPTER 14

Nursing Management During Labor and Birth

SECTION I: LEARNING OBJECTIVES

1. Define the key terms related to the labor and birth process.

2. Select the measures used to evaluate maternal status during labor and birth.

3. Compare and contrast the advantages and disadvantages of external and internal fetal monitoring, including the appropriate use for each.

4. Choose appropriate nursing interventions to address nonreassuring fetal heart rate patterns.

5. Outline the nurse's role in fetal assessment.

6. Explain the various comfort-promotion and pain-relief strategies used during labor and birth.

7. Summarize the assessment data collected on admission to the perinatal unit.

8. Plan the ongoing assessment involved in each stage of labor and birth.

9. Delineate the nurse's role throughout the labor and birth process.

SECTION II: ASSESSING YOUR UNDERSTANDING

Activity A *Fill in the blanks.*

1. _____ comfort measures are usually simple, safe, effective, and inexpensive to use.

2. If the woman is a diabetic, it is critical to alert the newborn nursery of potential _____ in the newborn.

3. If the nitrazine test is inconclusive, an additional test, called the _____ test, can be used to confirm rupture of membranes.

4. The nurse reviews the prenatal record to identify risk factors that may contribute to a decrease in _____ circulation during pregnancy and/or labor.

5. The _____ spines serve as landmarks for estimating the descent of the fetal presenting part and have been designated as zero station.

6. The primary power of labor is _____ contractions, which are involuntary.

7. The _____ is placed over the uterine fundus in the area of greatest contractility to electronically monitor uterine contractions.

8. _____ describes the irregular variations or absence of FHR due to erroneous causes on the fetal monitor record.

9. Baseline variability represents the interplay between the _____ and sympathetic nervous systems.

10. Fetal _____ are transitory increases in the FHR above the baseline that are associated with sympathetic nervous stimulation.

Activity B *Consider the following figure.*

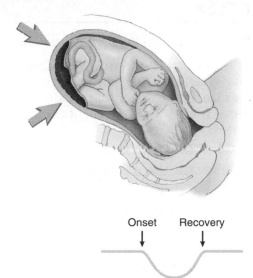

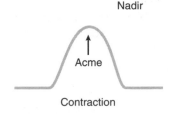

Onset   Recovery

Nadir

Acme

Contraction

1. a. Identify the FHR pattern shown in the image.

_____

_____

b. What causes this FHR pattern?

_____

_____

Activity C *Match the extent of the lacerations in Column A with their depths in Column B.*

Column A

_____ **1.** First-degree laceration

_____ **2.** Second-degree laceration

_____ **3.** Third-degree laceration

_____ **4.** Fourth-degree laceration

Column B

a. Through the anal sphincter muscle

b. Through the muscles of the perineal body

c. Through the skin

d. Through the anterior rectal wall

Activity D *Put the items in correct sequence by writing the letters in the boxes provided below.*

1. Given below, in random order, are nursing interventions during various stages of labor and birth. Arrange them in the correct order.

a. Check the fundus to ensure that it is firm (size and consistency of a grapefruit), located in the midline and below the umbilicus

b. Ascertain whether the woman is in true or false labor

c. Position the woman and cleanse the vulva and perineal areas

d. Check for lengthening of umbilical cord protruding from vagina

e. Check for crowning, low grunting sounds from the woman, and increase in blood-tinged show

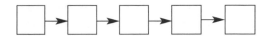

Activity E *Briefly answer the following.*

1. What information should a nurse include when taking the maternal health history?

_____

_____

_____

2. What does the Apgar score assess?

_____

_____

_____

3. What is the purpose of vaginal examination during maternal assessment?

_____

_____

_____

4. What are the advantages and disadvantages of continuous electronic fetal monitoring?

_____

_____

_____

5. What are the typical signs of the second stage of labor?

_____

_____

_____

6. What are the ideal positions for the second stage of labor?

_____

_____

_____

SECTION III: APPLYING YOUR KNOWLEDGE

Activity F *Consider this scenario and answer the questions.*

1. Susan, a pregnant client, has been admitted to the health care facility because she is in labor. The nurse is prepared to do maternal assessment during labor and delivery. Susan informs the nurse that there is no vaginal bleeding.

a. What nursing intervention should the nurse perform?

_____

_____

_____

b. What is the purpose of vaginal examination during maternal assessment?

_____

_____

_____

c. What is the procedure for conducting vaginal examination?

_____

_____

_____

SECTION IV: PRACTICING FOR NCLEX

Activity G *Answer the following questions.*

1. It is the nurse's first meeting with a pregnant client. What is the first point that the nurse needs to ascertain as part of the admission assessment to check if the client needs to be admitted?

a. Whether the client is in true or false labor

b. Whether the client is pregnant for the first time

c. Whether the client is addicted to drugs

d. Whether the client has a history of drug allergy

2. A nurse is assigned to conduct an admission assessment on the phone for a pregnant client. Which of the following information should the nurse obtain from the client? Select all that apply.

a. Estimated due date

b. History of drug abuse

c. Characteristics of contractions

d. Appearance of vaginal blood

e. History of drug allergy

3. A nurse is caring for a pregnant client who is in the active phase of labor. At what interval should the nurse monitor the client for maternal vital signs?

a. Every 15–30 minutes

b. Every 30 minutes

c. Every 30–60 minutes

d. Every 4 hours

4. A nurse is required to obtain the fetal heart rate (FHR) for a pregnant client. If the presentation is cephalic, which maternal site should the nurse monitor to hear the FHR clearly?

a. Lower quadrant of maternal abdomen

b. At the level of the maternal umbilicus

c. Above the level of maternal umbilicus

d. Just below the maternal umbilicus

5. Which of the following does fetal pulse oximetry help measure?
   a. Weight of the fetus
   b. Fetal blood pH
   c. Fetal oxygen saturation
   d. Fetal position

6. A client in labor is administered lorazepam to help her relax enough so that she can participate effectively during her labor process rather than fighting against it. Which of the following is an adverse effect of the drug that the nurse should monitor for?
   a. Increased sedation
   b. Newborn respiratory depression
   c. Nervous system depression
   d. Decreased alertness

7. A pregnant client with a history of spinal injury is being prepared for a cesarean birth. Which of the following methods of anesthesia is to be administered to the client?
   a. Local infiltration
   b. Epidural block
   c. Regional anesthesia
   d. General anesthesia

8. A pregnant client admitted to a health care center is in the latent phase of labor. How often should the nurse monitor the FHR with the Doppler during the latent phase?
   a. Every 30 minutes
   b. Every hour
   c. Every 15–30 minutes
   d. Continuously

9. During an admission assessment of a client in labor, the nurse observes that there is no vaginal bleeding yet. What nursing intervention is appropriate in the absence of vaginal bleeding when the client is in the early stage of labor?
   a. Monitor vital signs
   b. Assess amount of cervical dilation
   c. Obtain urine specimen for urinalysis
   d. Monitor hydration status

10. A pregnant client is admitted with vaginal bleeding. The nurse performs a nitrazine test to confirm that the membranes have rup-

tured. The nitrazine tape remains yellow to olive green, with pH between 5 and 6. What does this indicate?
   a. Membranes have ruptured
   b. Presence of amniotic fluid
   c. Presence of vaginal fluid
   d. Presence of excess blood

11. A nurse assisting a pregnant client during pregnancy is to monitor uterine contractions. Which of the following factors should the nurse assess to monitor uterine contraction? Select all that apply.
   a. Uterine resting tone
   b. Frequency of contractions
   c. Change in temperature
   d. Change in blood pressure
   e. Intensity of contractions

12. The nurse performing Leopold's maneuvers for a pregnant client explains to the client the purpose of the maneuvers. Which of the following is the purpose of Leopold's maneuvers? Select all that apply.
   a. Determining the presentation of the fetus
   b. Determining the position of the fetus
   c. Determining the lie of the fetus
   d. Determining the weight of the fetus
   e. Determining the size of the fetus

13. A nurse caring for a pregnant client in labor observes that the FHR is below 110. Which of the following interventions should the nurse perform? Select all that apply.
   a. Turn the client on her left side
   b. Reduce IV fluid rate
   c. Administer oxygen by mask
   d. Assess client for underlying causes
   e. Ignore questions from the client

14. The nurse caring for a client in preterm labor observes nonreassuring FHR patterns. Which of the following nursing interventions should the nurse perform?
   a. Application of vibroacoustic stimulation
   b. Tactile stimulation
   c. Administration of oxygen by mask
   d. Fetal scalp stimulation

15. A nurse is caring for a client administered an epidural block. Which of the following symptoms must the nurse monitor the client for?

    a. Respiratory depression

    b. Accidental intrathecal blockade

    c. Inadequate or failed block

    d. Postdural puncture headache

16. A client administered combined spinal-epidural analgesia is showing signs of hypotension and associated FHR changes. What interventions should the nurse perform to manage the changes?

    a. Assist client to a supine position

    b. Provide supplemental oxygen

    c. Discontinue IV fluid

    d. Turn client to her left side

17. A nurse is caring for a client administered general anesthesia for an emergency cesarean birth. What complications associated with general anesthesia should the nurse monitor for?

    a. Pruritus

    b. Uterine relaxation

    c. Inadequate or failed block

    d. Maternal hypotension

18. A pregnant client has opted for hydrotherapy for pain management during labor. Which of the following should the nurse consider when assisting the client during the birthing process?

    a. Initiate the technique only when the client is in active labor

    b. Do not allow the client to stay in the bath for long

    c. Ensure that the water temperature exceeds body temperature

    d. Allow the client into the water only if her membranes have ruptured

19. A nurse is teaching a couple about patterned breathing during their childbirth education. Which of the following techniques should the nurse suggest for slow-paced breathing?

    a. Inhale and exhale through the mouth at a rate of 4 breaths every 5 seconds

    b. Inhale slowly through nose and exhale through pursed lips

    c. Punctuated breathing by a forceful exhalation through pursed lips every few breaths

    d. Hold breath for 5 seconds after every three breaths

20. A pregnant client requires administration of an epidural block for management of pain during labor. Which of the following conditions should the nurse check for in the client before administering the epidural block? Select all that apply.

    a. Spinal abnormality

    b. Hypovolemia

    c. Varicose veins

    d. Coagulation defects

    e. Skin rashes or bruises

Postpartum Adaptations

SECTION I: LEARNING OBJECTIVES

1. Define the key terms bolded in this chapter.

2. Explain the systemic physiologic changes occurring in the woman after childbirth.

3. Identify the phases of maternal role adjustment as described by Reva Rubin.

4. Analyze the psychological adaptations occurring in the mother's partner after childbirth.

SECTION II: ASSESSING YOUR UNDERSTANDING

Activity A *Fill in the blanks.*

1. Within 10 days of birth, the fundus of the uterus usually cannot be palpated because it has descended into the true _____.

2. If retrogressive changes do not occur as a result of retained placental fragments or infection, _____ results.

3. _____ are the painful uterine contractions some women experience during the early postpartum period.

4. Increased prolactin levels and abundant milk supply, combined with inadequate emptying of the breast, may cause breast _____.

5. During pregnancy, stretching of the abdominal wall muscles occurs to accommodate the enlarging _____.

6. _____ acts so that milk can be ejected from the alveoli to the nipple.

7. For _____ women, menstruation usually resumes 7 to 9 weeks after giving birth.

8. _____ is the secretion of milk by the breasts.

9. _____ from the anterior pituitary gland, secreted in increasing levels throughout pregnancy, triggers synthesis and secretion of milk after giving birth.

10. The profuse _____ that is common during the early postpartum period is one of the most noticeable adaptations in the integumentary system and is a way of eliminating excess body fluids retained during pregnancy.

Activity B *Match the terms in Column A with their descriptions in Column B.*

Column A

____ 1. Engrossment

____ 2. Involution

____ 3. Lochia

____ 4. Puerperium

____ 5. Uterine atony

Column B

a. The discharge that occurs after birth

b. Encompasses the time after delivery as the woman's body begins to return to the prepregnant state

c. Allows excessive bleeding

d. The father's developing a bond with his newborn, which is a time of intense absorption, preoccupation, and interest

e. Involves three retrogressive processes, which are contraction of muscle fibers, catabolism, and regeneration of uterine epithelium

Activity C *Put the items in correct sequence by writing the letters in the boxes provided below.*

1. Lochia refers to the discharge that occurs after birth. Given below, in random order, are the three stages of lochia. Choose the correct sequence in which they appear after birth.

   a. Lochia alba

   b. Lochia rubra

   c. Lochia serosa

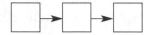

2. Given below, in random order, are the three stages a woman goes through immediately after she gives birth to a child. Choose the correct sequence in which they occur.

   a. Letting-go phase

   b. Taking-hold phase

   c. Taking-in phase

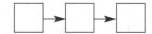

Activity D *Briefly answer the following.*

1. Explain why breastfeeding is not a reliable method of contraception.

   _____

   _____

   _____

2. Why are afterpains more acute in multiparous women?

   _____

   _____

   _____

3. What are the factors that facilitate uterine involution?

   _____

   _____

   _____

4. What are the factors that inhibit involution?

   _____

   _____

   _____

5. Why do women who have had cesarean births tend to have less flow of lochial discharge?

   _____

   _____

   _____

6. Why are afterpains usually stronger during breastfeeding? What can be done to reduce this discomfort?

   _____

   _____

   _____

SECTION III: APPLYING YOUR KNOWLEDGE

Activity E *Consider this scenario and answer the questions.*

1. A nurse is caring for two clients, one who is breastfeeding and has developed breast engorgement, and another who is not breastfeeding and has developed breast engorgement.

   a. What relief measures should the nurse suggest to resolve engorgement in the client who is breastfeeding?

   _____

   _____

   _____

   b. What relief measures should a nurse suggest for non-breastfeeding engorgement?

   _____

   _____

   _____

SECTION IV: PRACTICING FOR NCLEX

Activity F *Answer the following questions.*

1. A nurse is caring for a client in the postpartum period. Which of the following processes should the nurse identify as retrogressive processes involved in involution? Select all that apply.
   a. Contraction of muscle fibers
   b. Return of breasts to their prepregnancy size
   c. Catabolism, which reduces individual myometrial cells
   d. Regeneration of uterine epithelium
   e. Retention of urine

2. A client who gave birth about 12 hours ago informs the nurse that she has been voiding small amounts of urine frequently. The nurse examines the client and notes the displacement of the uterus from the midline to the right. What intervention should the nurse suggest or perform?
   a. Warm shower
   b. Good body mechanics
   c. Warm compress
   d. Catheterization

3. A client who has given birth a week ago complains to the nurse of discomfort when defecating and ambulating. The birth involved an episiotomy. Which of the following should the nurse suggest to the client to provide local comfort? Select all that apply.
   a. Maintain correct posture
   b. Use of warm sitz baths
   c. Use of anesthetic sprays
   d. Use of witch hazel pads
   e. Use good body mechanics

4. A nurse is caring for a client who has had a vaginal birth. The nurse understands that pelvic relaxation can occur in any woman experiencing a vaginal birth. Which of the following should the nurse recommend to the client to improve pelvic floor tone?
   a. Kegel exercises
   b. Witch hazel pads
   c. Good body mechanics
   d. Sitz baths

5. The nurse is caring for a client who had been administered an anesthetic block during labor. Which of the following are risks that the nurse should watch for in the client? Select all that apply.
   a. Incomplete emptying of bladder
   b. Bladder distention
   c. Ambulation difficulty
   d. Urinary retention
   e. Perineal laceration

6. A client who delivered a baby 36 hours ago informs the nurse that she has been passing unusually large volumes of urine very often. How should the nurse explain this to the client?
   a. Bruising and swelling of the perineum
   b. Swelling of tissues surrounding the urinary meatus
   c. Retention of extra fluids during pregnancy
   d. Decreased bladder tone due to anesthesia

7. A client complains to the nurse of pain in the lower back, hips, and joints 10 days after the birth of her baby. What instruction should the nurse give the client after birth to prevent low back pain and injury to the joints?
   a. Use anesthetic sprays
   b. Maintain correct position
   c. Practice Kegel exercises
   d. Apply ice

8. A concerned client tells the nurse that her husband, who was so excited about the baby before its birth, is apparently happy but seems to be afraid of caring for the baby. What suggestions should the nurse give to the client's husband to resolve the issue?
   a. Hold the newborn
   b. Speak to his friends
   c. Read up on parental care
   d. Speak to the physician

9. A client who gave birth five days ago complains to the nurse of profuse sweating during the night. What should the nurse recommend to the client in this regard?
   a. Use good body mechanics
   b. Use sitz baths
   c. Change her gown
   d. Practice Kegel exercises

10. A client is undergoing a routine check-up two months after the birth of her child. The nurse understands that the client is not practicing Kegel exercises. Which of the following should the nurse tell the client is caused by poor perineal muscular tone?

 a. Pain in the joints

 b. Pain in the lower back

 c. Urinary incontinence

 d. Postpartum diuresis

11. A breastfeeding client informs the nurse that she is unable to maintain her milk supply. What instructions should the nurse give to the client to improve milk supply?

 a. Take cold baths

 b. Apply ice to the breasts

 c. Empty the breasts frequently

 d. Perform Kegel exercises

12. A nurse is examining a client who underwent a vaginal birth 24 hours ago. The client tells the nurse that she is bleeding profusely. What explanation should the nurse give the client about lochia rubra?

 a. Discharge consists of mucus, tissue debris, and blood

 b. Discharge consists of leukocytes, decidual tissue, RBCs, and serous fluid

 c. Discharge consists of RBCs and leukocytes

 d. Discharge consists of leukocytes and decidual tissue

13. A nurse is caring for a client who gave birth a week ago. The client informs the nurse that she experiences painful uterine contractions when breastfeeding the baby. What should the nurse explain is the cause for such afterpains?

 a. Relaxin

 b. Progesterone

 c. Prolactin

 d. Oxytocin

CHAPTER 16

Nursing Management During the Postpartum Period

SECTION I: LEARNING OBJECTIVES

1. Define the key terms that are bolded throughout the chapter.

2. Categorize the parameters requiring assessment during the postpartum period.

3. Compare the bonding and attachment process.

4. Identify behaviors that enhance or inhibit the attachment process.

5. Outline nursing management for the woman and her family during the postpartum period.

6. Design the role of the nurse in promoting successful breastfeeding.

7. Plan areas of health education needed for discharge planning, home care, and follow-up.

SECTION II: ASSESSING YOUR UNDERSTANDING

Activity A *Fill in the blanks.*

1. The _____ is a plastic squeeze bottle filled with warm tap water that is sprayed over the perineal area after each voiding and before applying a new perineal pad.

2. Palpate the breasts for any nodules, masses, or areas of warmth, which may indicate a plugged duct that may progress to _____ if not treated promptly.

3. Elevations in blood pressure from the woman's baseline might suggest pregnancy-induced _____.

4. _____ is considered the fifth vital sign.

5. _____ hypotension can occur when the woman changes rapidly from a lying or sitting position to a standing one.

6. The top portion of the uterus, known as the _____, is assessed to determine uterine involution.

7. Women who experience _____ births will have less lochia discharge than those having a vaginal birth.

8. _____ is the process by which the infant's capabilities and behavioral characteristics elicit parental response.

9. _____ refers to the enduring nature of the attachment relationship.

10. Any discharge from the nipple should be described and documented if it is not _____, or foremilk.

Activity B *Match the terms in Column A with their descriptions in Column B.*

Column A

_____ **1.** Bonding

_____ **2.** Proximity

_____ **3.** Process of attachment

_____ **4.** Postpartum blues

Column B

a. Physical and psychological experience of the parents being close to their infant

b. Transient emotional disturbances

c. Development of a close emotional attachment to a newborn by the parents during the first 30 to 60 minutes after birth

d. Development of strong affectional ties between an infant and a significant other (e.g., mother, father, sibling, caretaker)

Activity C *Briefly answer the following.*

1. What does the postpartum assessment of the mother include?

_____

_____

_____

2. What nutritional recommendations can a nurse provide to a client during the postpartum period?

_____

_____

_____

3. What are the causes of postpartum stress?

_____

_____

_____

4. What are the postpartum danger signs?

_____

_____

_____

5. Discuss ways a nurse can model behavior to facilitate parental role adaptation and attachment during the postpartum period.

_____

_____

_____

6. What suggestions can a nurse provide to the parents to minimize sibling rivalry during the postpartum period?

_____

_____

_____

SECTION III: APPLYING YOUR KNOWLEDGE

Activity D *Consider this scenario and answer the questions.*

1. A nurse is caring for a client who has just delivered a healthy baby girl. The client is aware of the benefits of breastfeeding. She expresses her desire to breastfeed her newborn.

a. What assessments should the nurse perform in this regard?

_____

_____

_____

b. How often should the client breastfeed her infant during the postpartum period?

_____

_____

_____

SECTION IV: PRACTICING FOR NCLEX

Activity E *Answer the following questions.*

1. A nurse has been assigned to the care of a client who has just given birth. How frequently should the nurse perform the assessments during the first hour after delivery?
   a. Every 30 minutes
   b. Every 15 minutes
   c. After 60 minutes
   d. After 45 minutes

2. A nurse, assigned to check the pulse, discerns tachycardia in a postpartum client. Which of the following does it suggest?
   a. Pulmonary edema
   b. Atelectasis
   c. Excessive blood loss
   d. Pulmonary embolism

3. A client complains of uterine complications. Which of the following signs should the nurse look for while monitoring the uterus for uterine atony?
   a. Fundus feels firm
   b. Foul-smelling urine
   c. Purulent drainage
   d. Boggy or relaxed uterus

4. The nurse observes a two-inch lochia stain on the perineal pad of a postpartum client. Which of the following terms should the nurse use to describe the amount of lochia present?
   a. Light
   b. Scant
   c. Moderate
   d. Large

5. A nurse is caring for a client who has just had an episiotomy. The nurse observes that the laceration extends through the perineal area and continues through the anterior rectal wall. Which of the following classifications will the nurse use to describe the laceration?
   a. First-degree laceration
   b. Second-degree laceration
   c. Third-degree laceration
   d. Fourth-degree laceration

6. A nurse is required to apply ice packs to a client who has had a vaginal delivery. Which of the following interventions should the nurse perform to ensure that the client gets the optimum benefits of the procedure?
   a. Apply ice packs directly to the perineal area
   b. Apply ice packs for 40 minutes continuously
   c. Ensure ice pack is changed frequently
   d. Use ice packs for a week after delivery

7. Which of the following exercises should a nurse suggest to the client during the first day of postpartum?
   a. Abdominal exercises
   b. Buttock exercises
   c. Thigh-toning exercises
   d. Kegel exercises

8. A first-time mother is nervous about breastfeeding. Which of the following interventions should the nurse perform to reduce maternal anxiety about breastfeeding?
   a. Reassure the mother that some newborns "latch on and catch on" right away, and some newborns take more time and patience
   b. Explain that breastfeeding comes naturally to all mothers
   c. Tell her that breastfeeding is a mechanical procedure that involves burping once in a while and that she should try finishing it quickly
   d. Ensure that the mother breastfeeds the infant using the cradle method only

9. A client who has a breastfeeding infant complains of sore nipples. Which of the following interventions can the nurse do to alleviate the client's condition?
   a. Recommend a moisturizing soap to clean the nipples
   b. Encourage use of breast pads with plastic liners
   c. Offer suggestions based on observation to correct positioning or latching
   d. Fasten nursing bra flaps immediately after feeding

10. A client who has given birth is being discharged from the health care facility. She wants to know how safe it would be for her to have intercourse. Which of the following instructions should the nurse provide to the client regarding intercourse after childbirth?

    a. Avoid use of water-based gel lubricants

    b. Resume intercourse if bright-red bleeding stops

    c. Avoid performing pelvic floor exercises

    d. Use oral contraceptives for contraception

11. A client has been discharged from the maternity clinic after a cesarean delivery. Which of the following is the most appropriate time for scheduling a follow-up appointment for the client?

    a. Within 3 weeks of hospital discharge

    b. Between 4 and 6 weeks after hospital discharge

    c. Within 2 weeks of hospital discharge

    d. Within 1 week of hospital discharge

12. A client is Rh-negative and has given birth to an infant who is Rh-positive. Within how many hours should Rh immunoglobulin be injected in the mother?

    a. 72

    b. 75

    c. 78

    d. 80

13. A nurse is to care for a client during the postpartum period. The client complains of pain and discomfort in her breasts. What signs should a nurse look for to find out if the client has engorged breasts? Select all that apply.

    a. Breasts are hard

    b. Breasts are tender

    c. Nipples are fissured

    d. Nipples are cracked

    e. Breasts are taut

14. A nurse is assessing a client during the postpartum period. Which of the following indicate normal postpartum adjustment? Select all that apply.

    a. Abdominal pain

    b. Active bowel sounds

    c. Tender abdomen

    d. Passing gas

    e. Nondistended abdomen

15. Which of the following interventions should the nurse perform to ensure that the nutritional requirements of newborn infants are met? Select all that apply.

    a. Give infants water and other foods to balance nutritional needs

    b. Show mothers how to initiate breastfeeding within 30 minutes of birth

    c. Encourage breastfeeding of the newborn infant on demand

    d. Provide breastfeeding infants with pacifiers

    e. Place baby in uninterrupted skin-to-skin contact with the mother

CHAPTER 17

Newborn Adaptation

SECTION I: LEARNING OBJECTIVES

1. Define the key terms.

2. Identify the major changes in body systems that occur as the newborn adapts to extrauterine life.

3. Enumerate the primary challenges faced by the newborn during the adaptation to extrauterine life.

4. Explain the three behavioral patterns of newborn behavioral adaptation.

5. Distinguish the five typical behavioral responses of the newborn.

SECTION II: ASSESSING YOUR UNDERSTANDING

Activity A *Fill in the blanks.*

1. _____ is the newborn's ability to process and respond to visual and auditory stimuli.

2. A _____ is an involuntary muscular response to a sensory stimulus.

3. The immune system's responses may be natural or _____.

4. _____ is the first stool passed by the newborn, which is composed of amniotic fluid, shed mucosal cells, intestinal secretions, and blood.

5. Human milk provides a passive mechanism to protect the newborn against the dangers of a deficient _____ defense system.

6. At birth, the pH of the stomach contents is mildly acidic, reflecting the pH of the _____ fluid.

7. _____ refers to the yellowing of the skin, sclera, and mucous membranes as a result of increased bilirubin blood levels.

8. The source of bilirubin in the newborn is the _____ of erythrocytes.

9. Newborn iron stores are determined by total body _____ content and length of gestation.

10. The primary body temperature regulators are located in the _____ and the central nervous system.

Activity B *Match the blood-supplying structures in Column A with their corresponding functions in Column B.*

Column A	Column B
____ 1. Umbilical vein	a. Allows majority of the umbilical vein blood to bypass liver and merge with blood moving through the vena cava, bringing it to the heart sooner
____ 2. Ductus venosus	
____ 3. Foramen ovale	
____ 4. Ductus arteriosus	b. Connects pulmonary artery to the aorta, which allows bypassing of the pulmonary circuit

c. Allows more than half the blood entering the right atrium to cross immediately to the left atrium

d. Carries oxygenated blood from placenta to

Activity C *Briefly answer the following.*

1. What is a newborn's response to auditory and visual stimuli?

_____

_____

_____

2. What are the expected neurobehavioral responses of the newborn?

_____

_____

_____

3. What events must occur before a newborn's lungs can maintain respiratory function?

_____

_____

_____

4. How is the amniotic fluid removed from the lungs of a newborn?

_____

_____

_____

5. What signs of abnormality should a nurse observe in a newborn's respiration?

_____

_____

_____

6. What are the nursing interventions that may help minimize regurgitation?

_____

_____

_____

SECTION III: APPLYING YOUR KNOWLEDGE

Activity D *Consider this scenario and answer the questions.*

1. A newborn is under the observation of a nurse in a health care facility. The child is crying and its heartbeat has increased. Usually, heartbeats are highest after birth and reach a plateau within a week after birth. During the first few minutes after birth, a newborn's heart rate is approximately 120 to 180 bpm. Thereafter, the heart rate begins to decrease to somewhere between 120 and 130 bpm.

a. What are the factors that increase the heart rate and blood pressure in a newborn?

_____

_____

_____

b. What are the factors that affect the hematologic values of a newborn?

_____

_____

_____

c. What are the benefits of delayed cord clamping after birth?

_____

_____

_____

SECTION IV: PRACTICING FOR NCLEX

Activity E *Answer the following questions.*

1. A client delivers a newborn in a local health care facility. What guidance should the nurse give to the client before discharge regarding care of the newborn at home?

a. Ensure cool air is circulating over the newborn to ward off the heat

b. Keep the newborn wrapped in a blanket, with a cap on its head

   c. Hold the newborn close to the body after taking a shower

   d. Refrain from using clothing and blankets in the crib

2. A nurse is explaining the benefits of breast-feeding to a client who has just delivered. Which of the following immunoglobulins does breast milk contain that boost a newborn's immune system as opposed to formula?

   a. IgA

   b. IgD

   c. IgE

   d. IgM

3. Which of the following are factors that increase the risk of overheating in a newborn? Select all that apply.

   a. Limited sweating ability

   b. Underdeveloped lungs

   c. Too-warm crib

   d. Limited insulation

   e. Lack of brown fat

4. A two-month-old infant is admitted to a local health care facility after experiencing heat loss. Which of the following manifestations should the nurse observe in the infant in order to confirm the occurrence of cold stress?

   a. Change in color of the urine

   b. Increase in the body temperature

   c. Lethargy and hypotonia

   d. Change in the color of the skin

5. Which of the following is a risk factor for the development of jaundice in a newborn?

   a. Formula feeding

   b. Oxytocin dosage

   c. Female gender

   d. Hepatitis A vaccine

6. Which of the following possibilities should a nurse keep in mind while administering IV therapy to a newborn?

   a. Heart rate increase

   b. Lower blood pressure

   c. Decrease in alertness

   d. Fluid overload

7. A client is worried that her newborn's stools are greenish, with an unpleasant odor. The newborn is being formula-fed. What instruction should the nurse give this client?

   a. Switch to breast milk

   b. Greenish stools with an unpleasant odor are normal

   c. Increase newborn's fluid intake

   d. Administer vitamin K supplements

8. A mother wants to know the caloric intake for her two-week-old newborn. Which of the following should the nurse suggest as the ideal caloric intake for a term newborn to regain lost weight?

   a. 80 kcal/kg/day

   b. 108 kcal/kg/day

   c. 150 kcal/kg/day

   d. 200 kcal/kg/day

9. Which of the following newborns are at a greater risk for cold stress?

   a. Preterm newborns

   b. Newborns being fed formula

   c. Post-term newborns

   d. Larger–than-average newborns

10. A client delivers a baby in the maternity unit of a local health care facility. Which of the following behaviors of the newborn should the nurse identify as the self-quieting ability of a newborn?

   a. Hand-to-mouth movements

   b. Movement of head and eyes

   c. Hyperactivity

   d. Movements of the legs

11. A nurse needs to check the blood glucose levels of a newborn under observation at a health care facility. When should the nurse check the newborn's initial glucose level?

   a. After the newborn has been fed

   b. 24 hours after admission to the nursery

   c. On admission to the nursery

   d. 5 hours after admission to the nursery

12. Which of the following interventions can a nurse perform to maintain a neutral thermal environment?

    a. Promote early breastfeeding

    b. Avoid skin-to-skin contact with the mother

    c. Keep the infant transporter cool

    d. Avoid bathing the newborn

13. A nurse is required to assess the temperature of a newborn, using a skin temperature probe. Which of the following points should the nurse keep in mind while taking the newborn's temperature?

    a. Ensure that the newborn is lying on his or her abdomen

    b. Place the temperature probe on the forehead

    c. Place the temperature probe over the liver

    d. Place the temperature probe on the buttocks

14. A nurse is assigned to care for an infant with high bilirubin levels. Which of the following symptoms of jaundice should the nurse monitor?

    a. Yellow mucous membranes

    b. Pinkish appearance of tongue

    c. Heart rate of 120 bpm

    d. Bluish skin discoloration

15. Which of the following is a characteristic of the stools of a breastfed newborn?

    a. Formed in consistency

    b. Completely odorless

    c. Firm in shape

    d. Yellowish gold color

CHAPTER 18

Nursing Management of the Newborn

SECTION I: LEARNING OBJECTIVES

1. Define the key terms bolded throughout the chapter.

2. Differentiate the assessments performed during the immediate newborn period.

3. Select the interventions appropriate to meet the immediate needs of the term newborn.

4. Distinguish the components of a typical physical examination of a newborn.

5. Identify common variations that can be noted during a newborn's physical examination.

6. Categorize common concerns regarding the newborn and appropriate interventions.

7. Compare the importance of the newborn screening tests.

8. Explain the common interventions appropriate during the early newborn period.

9. Delineate the nurse's role in meeting the newborn's nutritional needs.

10. Outline discharge planning content and education needed for the family with a newborn.

SECTION II: ASSESSING YOUR UNDERSTANDING

Activity A *Fill in the blanks.*

1. The _____ score is used to evaluate newborns at 1 minute and 5 minutes after birth.

2. _____ refers to the soft, downy hair on the newborn's body.

3. _____ babies are babies with placental aging who are born after 42 weeks.

4. Babies weighing more than the 90th percentile on standard growth charts are referred to as _____ for gestational age.

5. Vitamin K, a fat-soluble vitamin, promotes blood clotting by increasing the synthesis of _____ by the liver.

6. Persistent cyanosis of fingers, hands, toes, and feet with mottled blue or red discoloration and coldness is called _____.

7. _____ are unopened sebaceous glands frequently found on a newborn's nose.

8. _____ sign refers to the dilation of blood vessels on only one side of the body, giving the newborn the appearance of paleness on one side of the body and ruddiness on the other.

9. The _____ fontanel of the baby is diamond shaped and closes by age 18 to 24 months.

10. _____ is a localized effusion of blood beneath the periosteum of the skull of the newborn.

Activity B *Consider the following figures.*

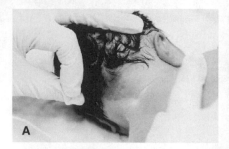

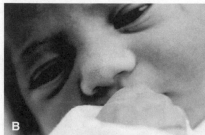

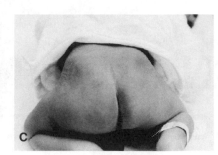

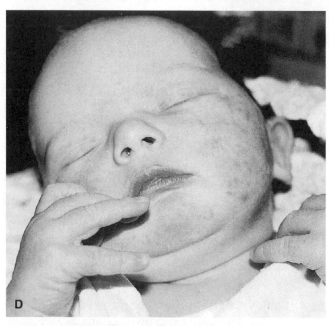

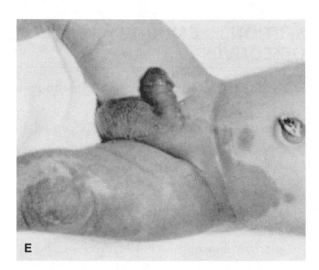

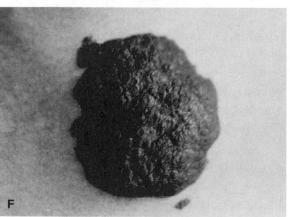

1. Identify the conditions in the figures.

_____

_____

2. What does the figure depict?

_____

_____

Activity C *Match the following anthropometric measurements of a term newborn in Column A with their appropriate value in Column B.*

Column A

____ **1.** Head circumference

____ **2.** Chest circumference

____ **3.** Weight

____ **4.** Length

Column B

a. 30–33 cm

b. 33–37 cm

c. 2500–4000 g

d. 45–55 cm

Activity D *Put the terms in correct sequence by writing the letters in the boxes provided below.*

1. Arrange the following reflexes in the correct order of their disappearance into adulthood.

a. Stepping

b. Babinski sign

c. Grasp

d. Rooting

e. Gag reflex

☐ → ☐ → ☐ → ☐ → ☐

Activity E *Briefly answer the following.*

1. How can a mother achieve the football hold position for breastfeeding?

_____

_____

_____

2. What is colostrum?

_____

_____

_____

3. What is the use of fiber optic pads in treatment of physiologic jaundice?

_____

_____

_____

4. How can a nurse test Moro's reflex?

_____

_____

_____

5. What is caput succedaneum?

_____

_____

_____

6. What is erythema toxicum?

_____

_____

_____

SECTION III: APPLYING YOUR KNOWLEDGE

Activity F *Consider this scenario and answer the questions.*

1. Karen, a first-time mother, is worried that her baby does not sleep properly and wakes up every two hours. Karen informs the nurse that she often brings the baby to her bed to nurse and falls asleep with the baby in her bed.

   a. What information should the nurse offer regarding the sleeping habits of newborns?

   _____

   _____

   _____

   b. What safety precautions should the mother take when putting the baby to sleep?

   _____

   _____

   _____

   c. What education should the nurse impart to Karen to discourage bed-sharing?

   _____

   _____

   _____

SECTION IV: PRACTICING FOR NCLEX

Activity G *Answer the following questions.*

1. The nurse caring for a newborn has to perform assessment at various intervals. When should the nurse complete the second assessment for the newborn?

   a. Immediately after birth, in the birthing area

   b. Within the first 2 to 4 hours, when newborn is in the nursery

   c. Before the newborn is discharged

   d. The day after the newborn's birth

2. A nurse is caring for a five-hour-old newborn. The physician has asked the nurse to maintain the newborn's temperature between 97.7° and 99.5°F (between 36.5° and 37.5°C). What nursing intervention should the nurse perform to maintain the temperature within the recommended range?

   a. Avoid measuring the weight of the infant, as scales may be cold

   b. Use the stethoscope over the baby's garment

   c. Place the newborn close to the outer wall in the room

   d. Place the newborn skin-to-skin with the mother

3. As a part of the newborn assessment, the nurse determines the skin turgor. Which of the following nursing interventions is relevant when observing the turgor of the newborn's skin?

   a. Pinch skin and note return to original position

   b. Examine for stork bites or salmon patches

   c. Check for unopened sebaceous glands

   d. Inspect for blue or purple splotches on buttocks

4. Which of the following information should the nurse give to a client who is breastfeeding her newborn regarding the nutritional requirements of newborns, as per the recommendations of AAP?

   a. Feed the infant at least 10 mL/kg of water daily

   b. Give iron supplements to the infant daily

   c. Give daily Vitamin D supplements for the first 2 months

   d. Ensure adequate fluoride supplementation

5. A first-time mother informs the nurse that she is unable to breastfeed her baby through the day, as she is usually away at work. She adds that she wants to express her breast milk and store it for her baby. What instruction should the nurse offer the woman to ensure the safety of frozen expressed breast milk?

   a. Use sealed and chilled milk within 24 hours

   b. Use frozen milk within 6 months of obtaining it

   c. Use microwave ovens to warm chilled milk

   d. Refreeze the used milk for later use

6. A nurse is educating the mother of a newborn about feeding and burping. Which of the following strategies should the nurse offer to the mother regarding burping?

   a. Hold the baby upright with the baby's head on her mother's shoulder

   b. Lay the baby on her back on her mother's lap

   c. Gently rub the baby's abdomen while the baby is in a sitting position

   d. Lay the baby on her mother's lap and give her frequent sips of warm water

7. The mother of a seven-month-old baby wishes to start the weaning process. What information should the nurse offer the client regarding introduction of solid foods?

   a. Introduce fruits after vegetables and eggs are introduced

   b. Introduce just one new single-ingredient food at a time to watch for allergies

   c. Coax the infant to eat if he or she is not willing to eat

   d. Avoid using a variety of solid foods in the diet

8. A nurse, while examining a newborn, observes salmon patches on the nape of the neck and on the eyelids. Which of the following is the most likely cause of the salmon patches?

   a. Concentration of pigmented cells

   b. Eosinophils reacting to environment

   c. Immature autoregulation of blood flow

   d. Concentration of immature blood vessels

9. A nurse is required to obtain the temperature of a healthy newborn who is placed in an ordinary crib. Which of the following is the most appropriate method for measuring a newborn's temperature?

   a. Tape electronic thermistor probe to the abdominal skin

   b. Obtain temperature orally

   c. Place electronic temperature probe in the midaxillary area

   d. Obtain temperature rectally

10. A nurse observes that a newborn has a 1-minute Apgar score of 5 points. What should the nurse conclude from the observed Apgar score?

    a. Severe distress in adjusting to extrauterine life

    b. Better condition of the newborn

    c. Moderate difficulty in adjusting to extrauterine life

    d. Abnormal central nervous system status

11. The mother of a newborn observes a diaper rash on her baby's skin. Which of the following should the nurse instruct the parent to prevent diaper rash?

    a. Expose the newborn's bottom to air several times a day

    b. Use plastic pants while bathing the infant

    c. Use products such as powder and items with fragrance

    d. Place the newborn's buttocks in warm water often

12. A nurse is caring for a newborn with transient tachypnea. What nursing interventions should the nurse perform while providing supportive care to the newborn? Select all that apply.

    a. Provide warm water to drink

    b. Provide oxygen supplement

    c. Massage the infant's back

    d. Ensure the newborn's warmth

    e. Observe respiratory status frequently

13. A nurse is caring for a newborn with hypoglycemia. What symptoms of hypoglycemia should the nurse monitor the newborn for? Select all that apply.

    a. Lethargy

    b. Low-pitched cry

    c. Cyanosis

    d. Skin rashes

    e. Jitteriness

14. A mother who is four days postpartum expresses to the nurse that her breast seems to be tender and engorged. What education should the nurse give to the mother to relieve breast engorgement? Select all that apply.

  a. Take warm-to-hot showers to encourage milk release

  b. Feed the newborn in the sitting position only

  c. Express some milk manually before breastfeeding

  d. Massage the breasts from the nipple toward the axillary area

  e. Apply warm compresses to the breasts prior to nursing

15. A nurse is performing detailed newborn assessment of a female baby. Which of the following observations indicate a normal finding? Select all that apply.

  a. Mongolian spots

  b. Enlarged fontanelles

  c. Swollen genitals

  d. Low-set ears

  e. Short, creased neck

CHAPTER 19

Nursing Management of Pregnancy at Risk: Pregnancy-Related Complications

SECTION I: LEARNING OBJECTIVES

1. Define the term *high-risk pregnancy*.

2. Explain common factors that might put a pregnancy at high risk.

3. Identify the causes of vaginal bleeding during early and late pregnancy.

4. Outline nursing assessment and management for the pregnant woman experiencing vaginal bleeding.

5. Develop a plan of care for the woman experiencing preeclampsia, eclampsia, and HELLP syndrome.

6. Explain the pathophysiology of polyhydramnios and subsequent management.

7. Select factors in a woman's prenatal history that place her at risk for premature rupture of membranes (PROM).

8. Formulate a teaching plan for maintaining the health of pregnant women experiencing a high-risk pregnancy.

SECTION II: ASSESSING YOUR UNDERSTANDING

Activity A *Fill in the blanks.*

1. _____ is a decreased amount of amniotic fluid (<500 mL) between 32 and 36 weeks' gestation.

2. _____ is the presence of rhythmic involuntary contractions, most often at the foot or ankle.

3. The time interval from rupture of membranes to the onset of regular contractions is termed the _____ period.

4. Brisk reflexes, or _____, are a common presenting symptom of preeclampsia and are the result of an irritable cortex.

5. Rh _____ is a condition that develops when a woman with Rh-negative blood type is exposed to Rh-positive blood cells and subsequently develops circulating titers of Rh antibodies.

6. _____ twins develop when a single, fertilized ovum splits during the first 2 weeks after conception.

7. A foul odor of amniotic fluid indicates
_____.

8. A _____ abortion refers to the loss of a
fetus resulting from natural causes—that is,
not elective or therapeutically induced by a
procedure.

9. The most common cause for _____
trimester abortions is fetal genetic abnormalities, usually unrelated to the mother.

10. _____ hypertension is characterized by
hypertension without proteinuria after 20
weeks of gestation and a return of the blood
pressure to normal postpartum.

Activity B *Consider the following figures.*

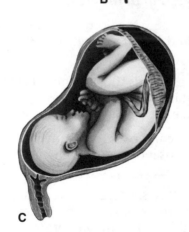

A

B

C

1. Identify the classifications of abruption placenta shown in the images.

_____

_____

Activity C *Match the following conditions
commonly associated with pregnancy-related
complications in Column A with their
definitions in Column B.*

Column A

___ **1.** Spontaneous
abortion

___ **2.** Ectopic
pregnancy

___ **3.** Gestational
trophoblastic
disease

___ **4.** Cervical
insufficiency

___ **5.** Placenta previa

Column B

a. Spectrum of neo-
plastic disorders
that originate in the
human placenta

b. Weak, structurally
defective cervix that
spontaneously di-
lates in the absence
of contractions in
the second
trimester, resulting
in the loss of the
pregnancy

c. Loss of an early
pregnancy, usually
before the 20th
week of gestation

d. Painless bleeding
condition that occurs
in the last two trime-
sters of pregnancy

e. Pregnancy in which
the fertilized ovum
implants outside
the uterine cavity

Activity D *Put the terms in correct sequence by
writing the letters in the boxes provided below.*

1. Given below, in random order, are the steps for
assessing the patellar reflex. Write the correct
sequence.

a. Using a reflex hammer or the side of the
hand, strike the area of the patellar tendon
firmly and quickly

b. Have the woman flex her knee slightly

c. Place the woman in the supine position

d. Repeat the procedure on the opposite leg

e. Note the movement of the leg and foot

f. Place a hand under the knee to support the
leg and locate the patellar tendon

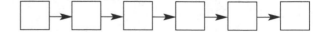

Activity E *Briefly answer the following.*

1. What are some possible complications of hyperemesis gravidarum?

_____

_____

_____

2. What are the conditions associated with early bleeding during pregnancy?

_____

_____

_____

3. What are the causes of ectopic pregnancies?

_____

_____

_____

4. What are the risk factors for hyperemesis gravidarum?

_____

_____

_____

5. What should a nurse include in prevention education for ectopic pregnancies?

_____

_____

_____

6. What is the Kleihauer–Betke test?

_____

_____

_____

SECTION III: APPLYING YOUR KNOWLEDGE

Activity F *Consider this scenario and answer the questions.*

1. The Labor and Birth triage nurse is admitting Jenna. By completing Jenna's history, the nurse learns that she is a single, 17-year-old African-American, G-3 P-0020, who registered for prenatal care at the local clinic at 16 weeks. Her prenatal course has been unremarkable except for a urinary tract infection at 22 weeks that was treated with antibiotics. She did not return to the clinic for a follow-up urine culture following treatment. She is presenting at the hospital now, at 26 weeks, complaining of lower backache, cramping, and malaise. She reports to the nurse that she feels normal fetal movement and denies vaginal bleeding or discharge. She states that she feels her uterus "balling up" every 5–10 minutes. This has been going on all day, even after she came home from school and rested. The external fetal monitor, tocodynamometer, and ultrasound are applied to Jenna. The nurse's initial assessment indicates Jenna having contractions every 4–5 minutes that last 30–40 seconds, and the nurse palpates the contractions as mild.

a. Name the symptoms that indicate preterm labor and birth.

_____

_____

_____

b. The nurse caring for Jenna must ensure that she receives basic information about preterm labor, including information about harmful lifestyles, the signs of genitourinary infections, and preterm labor. What information should the nurse provide to Jenna to help better educate her in prevention strategies?

_____

_____

_____

_____

SECTION IV: PRACTICING FOR NCLEX

Activity G *Answer the following questions.*

1. A pregnant client with hyperemesis gravidarum needs advice on how to minimize nausea and vomiting. Which of the following instructions should a nurse give this client?

a. Lie down or recline for at least two hours after eating

b. Avoid dry crackers, toast and soda

c. Eat small, frequent meals throughout the day

d. Decrease intake of carbonated beverages

2. When caring for a client with premature rupture of membranes (PROM), the nurse observes an increase in the client's pulse. What does this increase in pulse indicate?

   a. Infection

   b. Preterm labor

   c. Cord compression

   d. Respiratory distress syndrome

3. A nurse is caring for a client who has just undergone delivery. What is the best method for the nurse to assess this client for postpartum hemorrhage?

   a. By assessing skin turgor

   b. By assessing blood pressure

   c. By frequently assessing uterine involution

   d. By monitoring hCG titers

4. A nurse is monitoring a client with premature rupture of membranes (PROM) who is in labor and observes meconium in the amniotic fluid. What does this indicate?

   a. Cord compression

   b. Fetal distress related to hypoxia

   c. Infection

   d. CNS involvement

5. The nurse is caring for a pregnant client with severe preeclampsia. Which of the following nursing interventions should a nurse perform to institute and maintain seizure precautions in this client?

   a. Provide a well-lit room

   b. Keep head of bed slightly elevated

   c. Place the client in a supine position

   d. Keep the suction equipment readily available

6. A client with preeclampsia is receiving magnesium sulfate to suppress or control seizures. Which of the following nursing interventions should a nurse perform to determine the effectiveness of therapy?

   a. Assess deep tendon reflexes

   b. Monitor intake and output

   c. Assess client's mucous membrane

   d. Assess client's skin turgor

7. A nurse is assessing pregnant clients for the risk of placenta previa. Which of the following clients faces the greatest risk for this condition?

   a. A 23-year-old client

   b. A client with a history of alcohol ingestion

   c. A client with a structurally defective cervix

   d. A client who had undergone a myomectomy to remove fibroids

8. A client is seeking advice for his pregnant wife, who is experiencing mild elevations in blood pressure. In which of the following positions should a nurse recommend the pregnant client rest?

   a. Supine position

   b. Lateral recumbent position

   c. Left lateral lying position

   d. Head of the bed slightly elevated

9. A nurse is caring for a client with hyperemesis gravidarum. Which of the following should be the first choice for fluid replacement for this client?

   a. Total parenteral nutrition

   b. IV fluids and antiemetics

   c. Percutaneous endoscopic gastrostomy

   d. 5% dextrose in lactated Ringer's solution with vitamins and electrolytes

10. A nurse has been assigned to assess a pregnant client for abruptio placenta. Which of the following is a classic manifestation of this condition that the nurse should assess for?

    a. Painless bright red vaginal bleeding

    b. Increased fetal movement

    c. "Knife-like" abdominal pain with vaginal bleeding

    d. Generalized vasospasm

11. A nurse is caring for a client undergoing treatment for ectopic pregnancy. Which of the following symptoms is observed in a client if rupture or hemorrhaging occurs before successfully treating the ectopic pregnancy?

    a. Phrenic nerve irritation

    b. Painless bright red vaginal bleeding

    c. Fetal distress

    d. Tetanic contractions

12. The nurse is required to assess a pregnant client who is complaining of vaginal bleeding. Which of the following assessments should be considered as a priority by the nurse?

    a. Monitoring uterine contractility

    b. Assessing signs of shock

    c. Determining the amount of funneling

    d. Assessing the amount and color of the bleeding

13. The nurse is required to monitor a pregnant client with fallopian tube rupture. Which of the following interventions should a nurse perform to identify development of hypovolemic shock in this client?

    a. Monitor the client's beta-hCG level

    b. Monitor the mass with transvaginal ultrasound

    c. Monitor the client's vital signs, bleeding

    d. Monitor the fetal heart rate

14. Which of the following instructions should a nurse give an Rh-negative nonimmunized client in her early weeks of pregnancy to prevent complications of blood incompatibility?

    a. Obtain RhoGAM at 28 weeks' gestation

    b. Consume a well-balanced, nutritional diet

    c. Avoid sexual activity until after 28 weeks

    d. Undergo periodic transvaginal ultrasound

15. A nurse is caring for a pregnant client with eclamptic seizure. Which of the following should the nurse know as a characteristic of eclampsia?

    a. Muscle rigidity is followed by facial twitching

    b. Respirations are rapid during the seizure

    c. Coma occurs after seizure

    d. Respiration fails after the seizure

16. A nurse is assessing a pregnant client with preeclampsia for suspected dependent edema. Which of the following is a characteristic of dependent edema?

    a. Dependent edema leaves a small depression or pit after finger pressure is applied to a swollen area

    b. Dependent edema occurs only in clients on bed rest

    c. Dependent edema can be measured when pressure is applied

    d. Dependent edema may be seen in the sacral area if the client is on bed rest

17. The nurse is assessing a client who is in her 24th week of pregnancy. The nurse knows that which of the client's presenting symptoms should be further assessed as a possible sign of preterm labor? Select all that apply.

    a. Increase in vaginal discharge

    b. Phrenic nerve irritation

    c. Rupture of membranes

    d. Uterine contractions

    e. Hypovolemic shock

18. A pregnant client is brought to the health care facility with signs of PROM (premature rupture of membranes). Which of the following are the associated conditions and complications of premature rupture of the membranes? Select all that apply.

    a. Prolapsed cord

    b. Abruptio placenta

    c. Spontaneous abortion

    d. Placenta previa

    e. Preterm labor

19. The nurse is required to assess a client for HELLP syndrome. Which of the following are the signs and symptoms of this condition? Select all that apply.

    a. Blood pressure higher than 160/110

    b. Epigastric pain

    c. Oliguria

    d. Upper right quadrant pain

    e. Hyperbilirubinemia

20. A nurse is monitoring a client with spontaneous abortion who has been prescribed misoprostol. The nurse knows that which of the following symptoms are common adverse effects associated with misoprostol? Select all that apply.

    a. Constipation

    b. Dyspepsia

    c. Headache

    d. Hypotension

    e. Tachycardia

Nursing Management of the Pregnancy at Risk: Selected Health Conditions and Vulnerable Populations

SECTION I: LEARNING OBJECTIVES

1. Identify at least two conditions present before pregnancy that can have a negative effect on a pregnancy.

2. Explain how a condition present before pregnancy can impact the woman physiologically and psychologically when she becomes pregnant.

3. Differentiate the nursing assessment and management for a pregnant woman with diabetes from that of a pregnant woman without diabetes.

4. Explore how congenital and acquired heart conditions can affect a woman's pregnancy.

5. Describe the nursing assessment and management of a pregnant woman with cardiovascular disorders and respiratory conditions.

6. Differentiate among the types of anemia affecting pregnant women in terms of prevention and management.

7. Describe the most common infections that can jeopardize a pregnancy and propose possible preventive strategies.

8. Explain the nurse's role in the prevention and management of adolescent pregnancy.

9. Identify the impact of pregnancy for a woman over the age of 35.

10. Develop a plan of care for the pregnant woman who is HIV-positive.

11. Examine the effects of substance abuse during pregnancy.

SECTION II: ASSESSING YOUR UNDERSTANDING

Activity A *Fill in the blanks.*

1. Human placental lactogen and growth hormone _____ increase in direct correlation with the growth of placental tissue, causing insulin resistance.

2. _____ diabetes of any severity increases the risk of fetal macrosomia.

3. Asthma is known as reactive _____ disease.

4. The _____ is the major site of involvement in the client with tuberculosis.

5. _____ results in reduced capacity of the blood to carry oxygen to the vital organs of the mother and fetus as a result of reduced quantities of RBCs or hemoglobin.

6. Vaginal and rectal specimens are cultured for the presence of a _____ .

7. _____ is a widespread parasitic infection caused by a one-celled protozoan.

8. _____ spans the time frame from the onset of puberty to the cessation of physical growth, roughly from 11 to 19 years of age.

9. _____ found in cigarettes causes vasoconstriction, transfers across the placenta, and reduces blood flow to the fetus, contributing to fetal hypoxia.

10. _____ is a psychoactive drug derived from the leaves of the coca plant, which grows in the Andes Mountains of Peru, Ecuador, and Bolivia.

Activity B *Consider the following figure.*

1. **a.** Identify the disorder shown in the image.

   _____

   _____

b. What are the characteristics of this disorder?

   _____

   _____

Activity C *Match the substances in Column A with their effect on pregnancy in Column B.*

Column A

____ **1.** Alcohol

____ **2.** Caffeine

____ **3.** Nicotine

____ **4.** Cocaine

____ **5.** Narcotics

____ **6.** Sedatives

Column B

a. Respiratory problems, feeding difficulties, disturbed sleep

b. Neonatal abstinence syndrome, preterm labor, IUGR, and preeclampsia

c. Vasoconstriction, tachycardia, hypertension, abruptio placenta, abortion, prune belly syndrome, IUGR

d. Reduced uteroplacental blood flow, decreased birth weight, abortion, prematurity, abruptio placenta

e. Decreased iron absorption; increased risk of anemia

f. Growth deficiencies, facial abnormalities, CNS impairment, behavioral disorders, and abnormal intellectual development

Activity D *Briefly answer the following.*

1. What are the complications in a pregnant client with hypertension?

   _____

   _____

   _____

2. What elements should be included during the physical examination of pregnant clients with asthma?

   _____

   _____

   _____

3. What are the factors the nurse should include in the teaching plan for a pregnant client with asthma?

_____

_____

_____

4. What is the procedure involved in the assessment of tuberculosis in pregnant clients?

_____

_____

_____

5. What are the developmental tasks associated with adolescent behavior?

_____

_____

_____

6. What are the effects of abuse of sedatives by the mother on her infant?

_____

_____

_____

SECTION III: APPLYING YOUR KNOWLEDGE

Activity E *Consider this scenario and answer the questions.*

1. A nurse is caring for a pregnant client with asthma. During pregnancy, the respiratory system of the client is affected by hormonal changes, mechanical changes, and prior respiratory conditions.

   a. When is a pregnant client likely to suffer an increase in asthma attacks?

   _____

   _____

   _____

   b. What does successful management of asthma in pregnancy involve?

   _____

   _____

   _____

c. What are the nursing interventions involved for a client with asthma during labor?

_____

_____

_____

SECTION IV: PRACTICING FOR NCLEX

Activity F *Answer the following questions.*

1. A nurse is caring for a pregnant client. The nurse learns from the report that the client is diabetic. Which of the following should the nurse identify as the effect of insulin resistance in the client?

   a. Hypertension

   b. Postprandial hyperglycemia

   c. Hypercholesterolemia

   d. Myocardial infarction

2. A nurse is caring for a pregnant client. During assessment, the nurse learns that the client has cardiovascular disease. Which of the following should the nurse identify as a major risk that can be faced by the offspring of the client?

   a. Respiratory distress syndrome

   b. Congenital varicella syndrome

   c. Sudden infant death syndrome

   d. Prune belly syndrome

3. What is the role of the nurse during the preconception counseling of a pregnant client with chronic hypertension?

   a. Stressing the avoidance of dairy products

   b. Stressing the positive benefits of a healthy lifestyle

   c. Stressing the increased use of vitamin D supplements

   d. Stressing regular walks and exercise

4. Which of the following should the nurse recognize as a symptom of cardiac decompensation?

   a. Swelling of the face

   b. Dry, rasping cough

   c. Slow, labored respiration

   d. Elevated temperature

5. A nurse is caring for a pregnant client with heart disease in a labor unit. Which of the following is the most important intervention for this client in the first 48 hours postpartum?
   a. Limiting sodium intake
   b. Inspecting the extremities for edema
   c. Ensuring that the client consumes a high-fiber diet
   d. Assessing for cardiac decompensation

6. A nurse is caring for a pregnant client with asthma. Which of the following interventions should the nurse include during physical examination of this client?
   a. Monitoring temperature frequently
   b. Assessing for signs of fatigue
   c. Monitoring frequency of headache
   d. Assessing for feeling nauseated

7. What important instruction should the nurse give a pregnant client with tuberculosis?
   a. Maintain adequate hydration
   b. Avoid direct sunlight
   c. Avoid red meat
   d. Wear light, cotton clothes

8. Which of the following should the nurse identify as a risk associated with anemia during pregnancy?
   a. Newborn with heart problems
   b. Fetal asphyxia
   c. Preterm birth
   d. Newborn with an enlarged liver

9. A nurse is caring for a client with cardiovascular disease who has just delivered. What nursing intervention should the nurse perform when caring for this client?
   a. Assess for shortness of breath
   b. Assess for possible fluid overload
   c. Assess for edema and note any pitting
   d. Auscultate heart sounds for abnormalities

10. A nurse is caring for a pregnant client who works at a daycare center and is in regular contact with children. What instructions should the nurse give this client in order to minimize risk of transmission of cytomegalovirus (CMV) to the fetus?
    a. Ensure thorough handwashing
    b. Seek consultation for antibiotics
    c. Avoid interacting with children
    d. Drink plenty of fluids

11. A nurse is caring for a pregnant adolescent client admitted to the maternity unit of a health care center. Which of the following is an important area that the nurse should address during assessment of the client?
    a. Sexual development of the client
    b. Whether sex was consensual
    c. Stress level of the client
    d. Knowledge of child development

12. A nurse is caring for a 40-year-old pregnant client. About which of the following should the nurse inform this client?
    a. Risk for coronary artery disease
    b. Avoid excessive exposure to sunlight
    c. Avoid consumption of poultry products
    d. Perform aerobic exercises daily

13. A nurse is caring for a pregnant client who is HIV-positive. Which of the following is the most important issue that the nurse should discuss with the client?
    a. Relationship with the spouse
    b. Physical contact with infant
    c. Visiting crowded places
    d. Avoidance of breastfeeding

14. A nurse is caring for a pregnant client who admits to occasional substance abuse. Which risk factor associated with substance abuse during pregnancy should the nurse caution the client about?
    a. Post-term birth
    b. High levels of anxiety
    c. Stillbirth
    d. Transient tachypnea of the newborn

15. A nurse is caring for a pregnant client. The initial interview reveals that the client is accustomed to drinking coffee at regular intervals. What possible effect of maternal coffee consumption during pregnancy should the nurse make the client aware of?
    a. Increased risk of heart disease
    b. Increased risk of anemia
    c. Increased risk of rickets
    d. Increased risk of scurvy

16. The nurse is caring for a pregnant client whose Kardex indicates that she is fond of meat, works with children, and has a pet cat. Which of the following instructions should the nurse give this client to prevent toxoplasmosis? Select all that apply.

    a. Eat meat cooked to 160°F

    b. Avoid cleaning the cat's litter box

    c. Keep the cat outdoors at all times

    d. Feed the cat only uncooked meat

    e. Avoid outdoor activities such as gardening

17. A pregnant client has been diagnosed with gestational diabetes. Which of the following are risk factors for developing gestational diabetes? Select all that apply.

    a. Maternal age less than 18 years

    b. Genitourinary tract abnormalities

    c. Obesity

    d. Hypertension

    e. Previous LGA infant

18. A nurse is caring for a pregnant client with sickle cell anemia. What should the nursing care for the client include? Select all that apply.

    a. Teach the client meticulous handwashing

    b. Assess serum electrolyte levels of the client at each visit

    c. Instruct client to consume protein-rich food

    d. Assess hydration status of the client at each visit

    e. Urge the client to drink 8 to 10 glasses of fluid daily

19. A nurse is caring for a newborn with fetal alcohol spectrum disorder. What characteristic of the fetal alcohol spectrum disorder should the nurse assess for in the newborn?

    a. Small head circumference

    b. Decreased blood glucose level

    c. Poor breathing pattern

    d. Wide eyes

20. A nurse is documenting a dietary plan for a pregnant client with pregestational diabetes. What instructions should the nurse include in the dietary plan for this client?

    a. Include more dairy products in the diet

    b. Include complex carbohydrates in the diet

    c. Eat only two meals per day

    d. Eat at least one egg per day

Nursing Management of Labor and Birth at Risk

SECTION I: LEARNING OBJECTIVES

1. Define dystocia.

2. Identify the four major abnormalities or problems associated with dysfunctional labor patterns, giving examples of each problem.

3. Describe the nursing management for the woman with dysfunctional labor experiencing a problem with the powers, passenger, passageway, and psyche.

4. Develop a plan of care for the woman experiencing preterm labor.

5. Discuss the nursing assessment and management of the woman experiencing a post-term pregnancy.

6. Explain four obstetric emergencies that can complicate labor and birth, including appropriate management for each.

7. Compare and contrast the nursing management for the woman undergoing labor induction or augmentation versus forceps and vacuum–assisted birth.

8. Summarize the plan of care for a woman who is to undergo a cesarean birth.

9. Discuss the key areas to be addressed when caring for a woman who is to undergo vaginal birth after cesarean (VBAC).

SECTION II: ASSESSING YOUR UNDERSTANDING

Activity A *Fill in the blanks.*

1. Abnormal or difficult labor is known as _____.

2. _____ presentation is frequently associated with multifetal pregnancies and grand multiparity.

3. _____ maneuver is used to identify deviations in fetal presentation or position.

4. _____ drugs promote uterine relaxation by interfering with uterine contraction.

5. _____ are given to enhance fetal lung maturity between 24 weeks and 34 weeks of gestation.

6. Fetal _____, a glycoprotein produced by the chorion, is found at the junction of the chorion and deciduas.

7. _____ score helps to identify women who would be most likely to achieve a successful induction.

8. _____ dilators absorb endocervical and local tissue fluids; as they enlarge they expand the endocervix and provide controlled mechanical pressure.

9. An _____ involves inserting a cervical hook through the cervical os to artificially rupture the membranes.

10. _____ is produced naturally by the posterior pituitary gland and stimulates contractions of the uterus.

Activity B *Consider the following figures.*

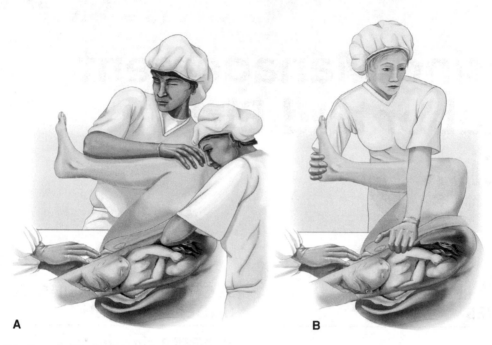

A   B

1. What do the figures depict?

_____

_____

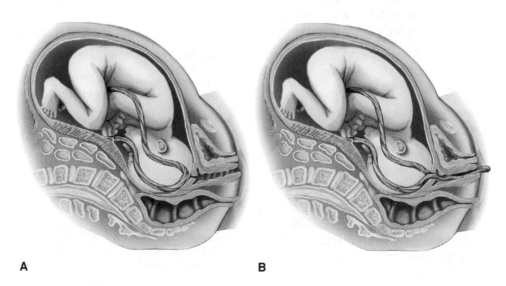

A   B

2. Identify the figures.

_____

_____

Activity C *Match the tests in Column A with their purposes in Column B.*

Column A

___ **1.** Ultrasound

___ **2.** Pelvimetry

___ **3.** Nonstress test

___ **4.** Phosphatidyl-glycerol (PG) level

___ **5.** Nitrazine paper and/or fern test

Column B

a. To rule out fetopelvic disproportion

b. To assess fetal lung maturity

c. To evaluate fetal size, position, and gestational age and to locate the placenta

d. To confirm ruptured membranes

e. To evaluate fetal well-being

Activity D *Put the terms in correct sequence by writing the letters in the boxes provided below.*

1. Given below, in random order, are steps for administering oxytocin. Choose the correct sequence.

a. Use an infusion pump on a secondary line connected to the primary infusion.

b. Prepare the oxytocin infusion by diluting 10 units of oxytocin in 1,000 mL of lactated Ringer's solution.

c. Perform or assist with periodic vaginal examinations to determine cervical dilation and fetal descent.

d. Start the oxytocin infusion in mU/min or mL/hour as ordered.

e. Monitor the characteristics of the FHR, including baseline rate, baseline variability, and decelerations.

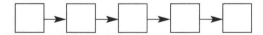

Activity E *Briefly answer the following.*

1. What are symptoms of preterm labor?

_____

_____

_____

2. What is cervical ripeness?

_____

_____

_____

3. What is uterine rupture?

_____

_____

_____

4. What are the indications and contraindications of amnioinfusion?

_____

_____

_____

5. What care should the nurse take when assessing the client for risk of cord prolapse?

_____

_____

_____

6. What are maternal and fetal complications in shoulder dystocia?

_____

_____

_____

SECTION III: APPLYING YOUR KNOWLEDGE

Activity F *Consider this scenario and answer the questions.*

1. Amnioinfusion is a technique in which a volume of warmed, sterile, normal saline or Ringer's lactate solution is introduced into the uterus through an intrauterine pressure catheter to increase the volume of fluid when oligohydramnios is present. It is used to change the relationship of the uterus, placenta, cord, and fetus to improve placental and fetal oxygenation. A nurse is caring for an antenatal mother who is advised to undergo amnioinfusion due to oligohydramnios. The nurse prepares the client for the procedure. What nursing interventions should the nurse follow when caring for the client to prevent maternal and fetal complications?

_____

_____

_____

SECTION IV: PRACTICING FOR NCLEX

Activity G *Answer the following questions.*

1. A nurse is assigned to care for a client who has to undergo a forceps and vacuum–assisted birth. The nurse understands that which of the following factors has contributed to a forceps and vacuum–assisted birth?
   a. A prolonged second stage of labor
   b. Oligohydramnios due to placental insufficiency
   c. Preterm labor with premature rupture of membranes
   d. Rupture of uterus

2. A nurse is assigned to care for a client who has been diagnosed with placental abruption. The nurse knows that which of the following could have led to placental abruption in the client?
   a. Obesity or excess weight gain
   b. Cardiovascular disease
   c. Gestational diabetes
   d. Gestational hypertension

3. A nurse is caring for a client who is experiencing acute onset of dyspnea and hypotension. The physician suspects the client has amniotic fluid embolism. Which of the following symptoms should a nurse monitor to verify the presence of this condition in the client?
   a. Cyanosis
   b. Arrhythmia
   c. Hyperglycemia
   d. Hematuria

4. A nurse is caring for obstetric clients. The nurse should be aware of which of the following as an indication for labor induction?
   a. Chorioamnionitis
   b. Complete placenta previa
   c. Abruptio placenta
   d. Transverse fetal lie

5. A nurse is caring for a client who is undergoing amnioinfusion. Which of the following should the nurse ensure to confirm that amnioinfusion is not contraindicated in this client?
   a. Client does not have uterine hypertonicity
   b. Client does not have an active genital herpes infection
   c. There are no signs of abruptio placentae
   d. Client does not have invasive cervical cancer

6. A client is experiencing shoulder dystocia during delivery. Which of the following should the nurse identify as risks to the fetus in such a condition?
   a. Extensive lacerations
   b. Bladder injury
   c. Infection
   d. Nerve damage

7. A full-term pregnant client is being assessed for induction of labor. Her Bishop score is less than six. Which of the following does it indicate?
   a. Cervical ripening method should be used
   b. A cesarean may be required
   c. Vaginal birth will be successful
   d. Labor will occur spontaneously

8. Which of the following postoperative interventions should a nurse perform when caring for a client who has undergone a cesarean section?
   a. Assess uterine tone to determine fundal firmness
   b. Delay breastfeeding the newborn for a day
   c. Ensure that the client does not cough or breathe deeply
   d. Avoid early ambulation to prevent respiratory problems

9. A client with full-term pregnancy who is not in active labor has been ordered oxytocin intravenously. Which of the following is a contraindication for oxytocin administration?

   a. Dysfunctional labor pattern

   b. Post-term status

   c. Prolonged ruptured membranes

   d. Overdistended uterus

10. A client who is in labor presents with shoulder dystocia of the fetus. Which of the following is an important nursing intervention?

    a. Assist with positioning the woman in squatting position

    b. Assess for complaints of intense back pain in first stage of labor

    c. Anticipate possible use of forceps to rotate to anterior position at birth

    d. Assess for prolonged second stage of labor with arrest of descent

11. A nurse is assessing the cause of multiple gestations in clients. Which of the following factors should the nurse assess as contributors to increased probability of multiple gestations?

    a. Infertility treatment

    b. Medications

    c. Advanced maternal age

    d. Adolescent pregnancies

12. A client is admitted to the health care facility with a gestational age of 42 weeks. The client is to undergo a cesarean section. Which of the following would be the fetal risk associated with post-term pregnancy?

    a. Underdeveloped suck reflex

    b. Congenital heart defects

    c. Intraventricular hemorrhage

    d. Cephalopelvic disproportion

13. A nurse is caring for a client who has been diagnosed with precipitous labor. For which of the following potential fetal complications should the nurse monitor as a result of precipitous labor?

    a. Facial nerve injury

    b. Cephalhematoma

    c. Intracranial hemorrhage

    d. Facial lacerations

14. A nurse is newly posted to the obstetric unit of the health care facility. Which of the following are the causes of intrauterine fetal demise in late pregnancy that the nurse should be aware of?

    a. Hydramnios

    b. Multifetal gestation

    c. Prolonged pregnancy

    d. Malpresentation

15. A nurse is caring for an antenatal mother diagnosed with umbilical cord prolapse. Which of the following should the nurse monitor for in a fetus in cases of umbilical cord prolapse?

    a. Fetal hypoxia

    b. Preeclampsia

    c. Coagulation defects

    d. Placental pathology

CHAPTER 22

Nursing Management of the Postpartum Woman at Risk

SECTION I: LEARNING OBJECTIVES

1. Define the major conditions associated with putting the postpartum woman at risk.

2. Explain the risk factors, assessment, preventive measures, and nursing management of common postpartum complications.

3. Differentiate the causes of postpartum hemorrhage based on the underlying pathophysiologic mechanisms.

4. Outline the role of the nurse in assessing and managing the care of a woman with a thromboembolic condition.

5. Discuss the nursing management of a woman who develops a postpartum infection.

6. Identify at least two affective disorders that can occur in women after birth, describing specific therapeutic management for each.

SECTION II: ASSESSING YOUR UNDERSTANDING

Activity A *Fill in the blanks.*

1. Failure of the uterus to contract and retract immediately after birth is called uterine _____.

2. _____ refers to the incomplete involution of the uterus, or its failure to return to its normal size and condition after birth.

3. In von Willebrand disease, there is a _____ in von Willebrand factor, which is necessary for platelet adhesion and aggregation.

4. A blood clot within a blood vessel is called a _____.

5. Obstruction of a blood vessel by a blood clot carried by the circulation from the site of origin is called _____.

6. _____ is an infectious condition that involves the endometrium, decidua, and adjacent myometrium of the uterus.

7. Inflammation of the breast is called _____.

8. Excessive blood loss that occurs within 24 hours after birth is termed _____ postpartum hemorrhage.

9. Placenta _____ is a condition in which the chorionic villi adhere to the myometrium, causing the placenta to adhere abnormally to the uterus and not separate and deliver spontaneously.

10. A prolapse of the uterine fundus to or through the cervix, so that the uterus is turned inside out after birth, is called uterine _____.

Activity B *Consider the following figures.*

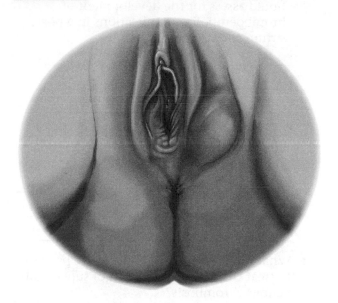

1. Identify the figure.

_____

_____

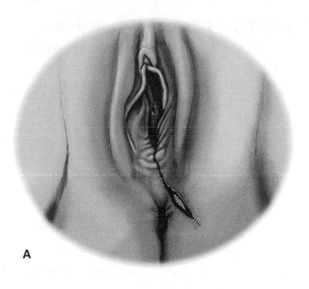

A

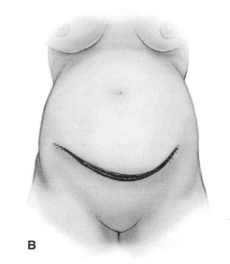

B

2. What does the figure depict?

_____

_____

Activity C *Match the following causes of postpartum hemorrhage in Column A with their appropriate intervention in Column B.*

Column A

_____ **1.** Uterine atony

_____ **2.** Retained placental tissue

_____ **3.** Lacerations or hematoma

_____ **4.** Bleeding disorder

Column B

a. Evacuation and oxytocics

b. Massage and oxytocics

c. Provide blood products

d. Surgical repair

Activity D *Briefly answer the following.*

1. What are the causes of overdistention of the uterus?

_____

_____

_____

2. What is idiopathic thrombocytopenia purpura?

_____

_____

_____

3. Which microorganisms are responsible for postpartum infections?

_____

_____

_____

4. What are baby blues?

_____

_____

_____

5. What are the symptoms of postpartum psychosis?

_____

_____

_____

6. What are the types of venous thrombosis?

_____

_____

_____

SECTION III: APPLYING YOUR KNOWLEDGE

Activity E *Consider this scenario and answer the questions.*

1. A 37-year-old client complains of calf pain following the vaginal delivery of her third child. On assessment, the nurse finds that the calf area is tender to the touch. The client is diagnosed with superficial venous thrombosis.

a. What are the risk factors for which a nurse should assess for the development of thromboembolic complications in a postpartum client?

_____

_____

_____

b. What nursing interventions should the nurse perform to prevent thromboembolic complications in clients?

_____

_____

_____

c. What interventions should a nurse perform to treat the client's condition of superficial venous thrombosis?

_____

_____

_____

_____

SECTION IV: PRACTICING FOR NCLEX

Activity F *Answer the following questions.*

1. A nurse is caring for a postpartum client who has a history of thrombosis during pregnancy and is at high risk of developing a pulmonary embolism. For which of the following should the nurse monitor the client to prevent occurrence of pulmonary embolism?

a. Sudden change in mental status

b. Difficulty in breathing

c. Calf swelling

d. Sudden chest pain

2. A nurse is caring for a client with deep vein thrombosis. Which of the following instructions should the nurse offer when caring for the client?

a. Avoid using compression stockings

b. Ensure long hours of bed rest

c. Avoid using products containing aspirin

d. Avoid use of oral contraceptives

3. A nurse is caring for a client with idiopathic thrombocytopenic purpura (ITP). Which of the following interventions should the nurse perform when caring for this client?

   a. Administer prescribed NSAIDs

   b. Administer platelet transfusions as ordered

   c. Refrain from administering oxytocics

   d. Continual firm massage of the uterus

4. Two weeks after a vaginal delivery, a client presents with low-grade fever. The client also complains of a loss of appetite and low energy levels. The physician suspects an infection of the episiotomy. Which of the following should the nurse assess to verify the presence of this condition?

   a. Foul-smelling vaginal discharge

   b. Sudden onset of shortness of breath

   c. Sudden change in mental status

   d. Apprehension and diaphoresis

5. A nurse is caring for a postpartum client diagnosed with von Willebrand disease. Which of the following should the nurse expect to find in the client?

   a. Prolonged bleeding time

   b. A fever of 100.4°F after the first 24 hours following childbirth

   c. Foul-smelling vaginal discharge

   d. Postpartum fundal height that is higher than expected

6. A nurse is assigned to care for a 38-year-old overweight client scheduled to undergo a cesarean section. The client is at an increased risk of thromboembolic complications. During assessment, what factor will help the nurse in the diagnosis of deep vein thrombosis of the leg?

   a. Sudden chest pain

   b. Dyspnea

   c. Tachypnea

   d. Calf tenderness

7. A nurse finds that a client is bleeding excessively after a vaginal delivery. Which of the following assessment findings would indicate retained placental fragments as a cause of bleeding?

   a. Soft and boggy uterus that deviates from the midline

   b. Firm uterus with trickle of bright-red blood in perineum

   c. Firm uterus with a steady stream of bright-red blood

   d. Large uterus with painless dark-red blood mixed with clots

8. A client has had a forceps delivery. This has resulted in lacerations and bleeding. How can a nurse identify if the bleeding is due to laceration?

   a. Look for a contracted uterus with vaginal bleeding

   b. Look for a subinvoluted uterus with vaginal bleeding

   c. Look for a boggy uterus with vaginal bleeding

   d. Look for an inverted uterus with vaginal bleeding

9. A nurse is caring for a client who has had a vaginal delivery two hours ago. Which of these can the nurse assess within the first few hours following delivery?

   a. Postpartal infection

   b. Postpartal blues

   c. Postpartal hemorrhage

   d. Postpartum depression

10. A nurse is a caring for a postpartum client. Which of the following instructions should the nurse provide to the client as precautionary measures to prevent thromboembolic complications?

    a. Avoid performing any deep-breathing exercises

    b. Try to relax with pillows under knees

    c. Avoid sitting in one position for long periods of time

    d. Refrain from elevating legs above heart level

11. A postpartum client had a difficult labor. Which of the following should the nurse monitor when evaluating the client for signs of hemorrhage?

    a. Decreased heart rate

    b. Increased urinary output

    c. Decreased blood pressure

    d. Increased body temperature

12. A postpartum client who was discharged home returns to the primary health care facility after two weeks with complaints of fever and pain in the breast. The client is diagnosed with mastitis. What education should the nurse give to the client for managing and preventing mastitis?

    a. Discontinue breastfeeding to allow time for healing

    b. Perform hand-washing before and after breastfeeding

    c. Avoid hot or cold compresses on the breast

    d. Discourage manual compression of breast for expressing milk

13. A nurse is caring for a client who has had an intrauterine fetal death with prolonged retention of the fetus. For which of the following factors should the nurse monitor in a client to assess for an increased risk of disseminated intravascular coagulation? Select all that apply.

    a. Hypertension

    b. Bleeding gums

    c. Tachycardia

    d. Acute renal failure

    e. Lochia less than usual

14. A client is in her seventh week of the postpartum period. She is experiencing bouts of sadness and insomnia. The client has developed postpartum depression. For which of the following signs and symptoms should a nurse monitor to verify this condition in the client? Select all that apply.

    a. Inability to concentrate

    b. Loss of confidence

    c. Manifestations of mania

    d. Decreased interest in life

    e. Bizarre behavior

15. A nurse is assessing a client with postpartal hemorrhage; the client is presently on IV oxytocin. Which of the following interventions should the nurse perform to evaluate the efficacy of the drug treatment? Select all that apply.

    a. Assess client's uterine tone

    b. Monitor client's vital signs

    c. Assess client's skin turgor

    d. Get a pad count

    e. Assess deep tendon reflexes

CHAPTER 23

Nursing Care of the Newborn With Special Needs

SECTION I: LEARNING OBJECTIVES

1. Explain factors that assist in identifying a newborn at risk due to variations in birth weight and gestational age.

2. Select contributing factors and common complications associated with dysmature infants and their management.

3. Compare and contrast a small–for-gestational-age newborn versus a large-for-gestational-age newborn and a post-term versus preterm newborn.

4. Identify associated conditions that affect the newborn with variations in birth weight and gestational age, including appropriate management.

5. Outline the nurse's role in helping parents experiencing perinatal grief or loss.

6. Integrate knowledge of the risks associated with late preterm births into nursing interventions, discharge planning, and parent education.

SECTION II: ASSESSING YOUR UNDERSTANDING

Activity A *Fill in the blanks.*

1. _____ is defined as a venous hematocrit of greater than 65%.

2. _____ feedings are used for compromised newborns to minimize energy expenditure from sucking during the feeding process.

3. A newborn who fails to establish adequate, sustained respiration after birth is said to have _____.

4. A _____ infant is born before the completion of 37 weeks.

5. One of the problems that affect the preterm infant's breathing ability and adjustment to extrauterine life includes an unstable chest wall, leading to _____.

6. A _____ newborn is an infant who is born from the first day of week 38 through 42 weeks.

7. _____ of prematurity is a potentially blinding eye disorder that occurs when abnormal blood vessels grow and spread through the retina, eventually leading to retinal detachment.

8. _____ assessment is considered the "fifth vital sign" and should be done as frequently as the other four vital signs.

9. Gestational age at birth is _____ correlated with the risk that the infant will experience physical, neurologic, or developmental sequelae.

10. Fetal growth is dependent on _____, placental, and maternal factors.

Activity B *Consider the following figure.*

1. **a.** Identify the figure.

   _____

   _____

   b. What is the purpose of the equipment depicted in the figure?

   _____

   _____

Activity C *Match the heat transfer mechanism in Column A with the ways to prevent heat loss in Column B.*

Column A

____ **1.** Convection

____ **2.** Conduction

____ **3.** Radiation

____ **4.** Evaporation

Column B

a. Warm everything the newborn comes in contact with

b. Provide insulation to prevent heat transfer

c. Avoid drafts near the newborn

d. Delay the first bath until the baby's temperature is stable

Activity D *Put the terms in correct sequence by writing the letters in the boxes provided below.*

1. Given below, in random order, are a set of actions performed when resuscitating the newborn. Rearrange them in the correct sequence.

   a. Administer epinephrine and/or volume expansion

   b. Position the head in a neutral position

   c. Clear the airway and stimulate breathing

   d. Provide warmth by placing the newborn under a radiant heater

   e. Dry the newborn thoroughly with a warm towel

   f. Provide ventilation and perform chest compressions

   □ → □ → □ → □ → □ → □

Activity E *Briefly answer the following.*

1. What are the physical characteristics of preterm newborns?

   _____

   _____

   _____

2. What are the signs of hypoglycemia in the newborn?

   _____

   _____

   _____

3. What is developmentally supportive care?

   _____

   _____

   _____

4. What are the risk factors to which a preterm infant is susceptible?

   _____

   _____

   _____

5. What are the characteristics of large-for-gestational-age newborns?

_____

_____

_____

6. What are the characteristics of post-term newborns?

_____

_____

_____

SECTION III: APPLYING YOUR KNOWLEDGE

Activity F *Consider this scenario and answer the questions.*

1. A nurse is caring for a preterm newborn who may not survive. The nurse is in the difficult situation of having to help the newborn's parents.

   a. How can a nurse help the parents in the detachment process in the case of a dying newborn?

   _____

   _____

   _____

   b. What are the nursing interventions when caring for a family experiencing a perinatal loss?

   _____

   _____

   _____

SECTION IV: PRACTICING FOR NCLEX

Activity G *Answer the following questions.*

1. A nurse is caring for an infant born with polycythemia. Which of the following is the most appropriate intervention that the nurse should perform for such an infant?

   a. Focus on decreasing blood viscosity by increasing fluid volume

   b. Check blood glucose within two hours of birth by reagent test strip

   c. Repeat screening every two to three hours or before feeds

   d. Focus on monitoring and maintaining blood glucose levels

2. Which of the following precautions should a nurse take to prevent infection in a newborn? Select all that apply.

   a. Avoid coming to work when ill

   b. Cover jewelry while washing hands

   c. Use sterile gloves for an invasive procedure

   d. Avoid using disposable equipment

   e. Monitor laboratory test results for changes

3. Which of the following interventions should a nurse perform, particularly when caring for a preterm infant?

   a. Rocking and massaging

   b. Swaddling and positioning

   c. Using minimal amount of tape

   d. Using distraction through objects

4. Which of the following is a risk to newborns because of meconium in the amniotic fluid?

   a. Bradycardia

   b. Perinatal asphyxia

   c. Acute respiratory complications

   d. Polycythemia

5. A nurse has placed an infant with asphyxia on a radiant warmer. Which of the following signs indicate that the resuscitation methods have been successful?

   a. 80 bpm pulse

   b. Tremors

   c. Bluish tongue

   d. Good cry

6. Which of the following interventions should a nurse perform to promote thermal regulation in a preterm newborn?

   a. Assess the newborn's temperature every five hours until stable

   b. Set the temperature of the radiant warmer at a fixed level

   c. Observe for clinical signs of cold stress such as weak cry

   d. Check the blood pressure of the infant every two hours

7. A nurse is caring for a preterm infant. Which of the following interventions should the nurse perform to prepare the preterm newborn's gut to overcome the many feeding difficulties?

    a. Administer vitamin D supplements

    b. Administer 0.5 mL of breast milk enterally

    c. Administer iron supplements

    d. Administer dextrose intravenously

8. A nurse is caring for an infant born with hypoglycemia. What care should the nurse administer to a newborn with hypoglycemia?

    a. Maintain fluid and electrolyte balance

    b. Give dextrose intravenously before oral feedings

    c. Place infant on radiant warmer immediately

    d. Focus on decreasing blood viscosity

9. Which of the following interventions should a nurse perform to promote nutrition and fluid balance in the post-term newborn?

    a. Measure weight once every two days

    b. Assess for increased muscle tone

    c. Assess for decrease in urinary output

    d. Monitor for fall in temperature for dehydration

10. Which of the following maternal factors should the nurse consider that could lead to a newborn's being "large for gestational age"? Select all that apply.

    a. Diabetes mellitus

    b. Postdates gestation

    c. Alcohol use

    d. Glucose intolerance

    e. Renal infection

11. Which of the following is a sign of polycythemia that the nurse should be aware of in an infant?

    a. Jaundice

    b. Restlessness

    c. Temperature instability

    d. Wheezing

12. A nurse observes that a newborn's blood glucose level is 23 mg/dL. Which of the following interventions should the nurse perform?

    a. Administer dextrose intravenously

    b. Monitor the infant's pulse closely

    c. Administer IV glucose immediately

    d. Place the infant on a radiant warmer

13. A nurse is caring for an infant born with a high bilirubin level. Which of the following measures should the nurse adopt to reduce the bilirubin level in the newborn? Select all that apply.

    a. Hydration

    b. Increase water intake

    c. Early feedings

    d. Administer vitamin supplements

    e. Phototherapy

14. Which of the following indicates meconium aspiration in a newborn?

    a. Bluish skin discoloration

    b. Listlessness or lethargy

    c. Stained umbilical cord

    d. Pink tongue

Nursing Management of the Newborn at Risk: Acquired and Congenital Newborn Conditions

SECTION I: LEARNING OBJECTIVES

1. Identify the most common acquired conditions affecting the newborn.

2. Describe the nursing management of a newborn experiencing respiratory distress syndrome.

3. Outline the birthing room preparation and procedures necessary to prevent meconium aspiration syndrome in the newborn at birth.

4. Discuss parent education for follow-up care needed by newborns with retinopathy of prematurity.

5. Differentiate risk factors for the development of necrotizing enterocolitis.

6. Explain the impact of maternal diabetes on the newborn and care needed.

7. Describe the assessment and intervention for a newborn experiencing substance withdrawal after birth.

8. Identify assessment and nursing management for newborns sustaining trauma and birth injuries.

9. Outline assessment, interventions, prevention, and management of hyperbilirubinemia in newborns.

10. Summarize the interventions appropriate for a newborn with neonatal sepsis.

11. Compare and contrast the four classifications of congenital heart disease.

12. Describe the major acquired congenital anomalies affecting the central nervous system, respiratory system, gastrointestinal system, genitourinary system, and musculoskeletal system that can occur in a newborn.

13. Discuss three inborn errors of metabolism.

14. Formulate a plan of care for a newborn with an acquired or congenital condition.

15. Discuss the importance of parental participation in care of the newborn with a congenital or acquired condition, including the nurse's role in facilitating parental involvement.

SECTION II: ASSESSING YOUR UNDERSTANDING

Activity A *Fill in the blanks.*

1. An _____ is a defect of the umbilical ring that allows evisceration of abdominal contents into an external peritoneal sac.

2. _____ is a subperiosteal collection of blood secondary to the rupture of blood vessels between the skull and periosteum.

3. _____ is a condition in which total serum bilirubin level is above 5 mg/dL and exhibited as jaundice.

4. Presence of bacterial, fungal, or viral microorganisms or their toxins in blood or other tissues in newborns is known as neonatal _____.

5. _____ is a synthetic opiate narcotic that is used primarily as maintenance therapy for heroin addiction.

6. Immune hydrops is a severe form of _____ disease of the newborn that occurs when pathologic changes develop in the organs of the fetus secondary to severe anemia.

7. For the newborn with jaundice, regardless of its etiology, _____ is used to convert unconjugated bilirubin to the less toxic water-soluble form that can be excreted.

8. _____ is a herniation of abdominal contents through an abdominal wall defect.

9. Failure to establish adequate, sustained respiration after birth is known as neonatal _____.

10. _____ is a preventable neurologic disorder characterized by encephalopathy, motor abnormalities, hearing and vision loss, and death.

11. In bronchopulmonary dysplasia high inspired oxygen concentrations cause an _____ process in the lungs that leads to parenchymal damage.

12. A _____ shunt is inserted from the ventricle in the brain and threaded down into the peritoneal cavity to allow drainage of excess CSF.

Activity B *Consider the following figures and answer the questions.*

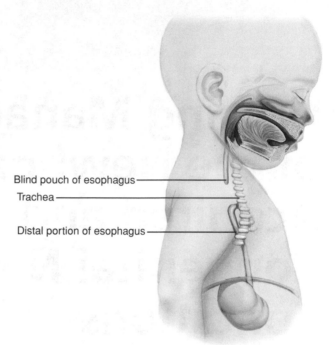

Blind pouch of esophagus

Trachea

Distal portion of esophagus

1. Identify the congenital condition shown in the image.

   _____

   _____

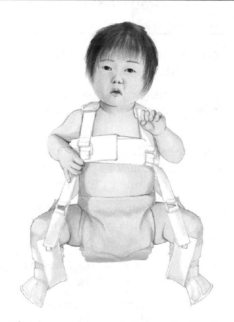

2. Identify the equipment shown in the image. Discuss its use.

   _____

   _____

Activity C

I. Match the commonly abused substances in Column A with their effects on newborns in Column B.

Column A

_____ **1.** Marijuana

_____ **2.** Cocaine

_____ **3.** Methamphetamines

_____ **4.** Heroin

Column B

a. Altered responses to visual stimuli, sleep-pattern abnormalities, photophobia

b. Frantic fist sucking, high-pitched cry, and significant lassitude

c. Stiff and hyper-extended positioning, limb defects, ambiguous genitalia

d. Smaller head circumference, piercing cry, genitourinary tract abnormalities

c. Vomiting, hypo-glycemia, liver damage, hyper-bilirubinemia, poor weight gain, cataracts, frequent infections

d. Newborns appear normal at birth but by six months of age signs of slow mental development evident

Activity D _Briefly answer the following._

1. What are the characteristics of an infant born to a diabetic mother?

_____

_____

_____

2. What are the most common types of malformations in infants of diabetic mothers?

_____

_____

_____

3. What does the treatment of infants born to diabetic mothers focus on?

_____

_____

_____

II. Match the inborn errors of metabolism in Column A with their clinical picture in Column B.

Column A

_____ **1.** Phenylketonuria (PKU)

_____ **2.** Maple syrup urine disease (MSUR)

_____ **3.** Galactosemia

_____ **4.** Congenital hypothyroidism

Column B

a. Large protruding tongue, slow reflexes, distended abdomen, large, open posterior fontanel, constipation, hypothermia, poor feeding, hoarse cry, dry skin, coarse hair, goiter, and jaundice

b. Lethargy, poor feeding, vomiting, weight loss, seizures, shrill cry, shallow respirations, loss of reflexes, coma

4. What are the causes of birth trauma?

_____

_____

_____

5. What is meconium aspiration syndrome?

_____

_____

_____

6. What is periventricular–intraventricular hemorrhage?

_____

_____

_____

7. What are the goals of therapy for a newborn with bladder exstrophy?

_____

_____

_____

8. As a nurse, how would you promote bonding between a newborn with a cleft lip and palate and its parents?

_____

_____

_____

SECTION III: APPLYING YOUR KNOWLEDGE

Activity E *Consider the scenario and answer the questions.*

A pregnant client visits a health care facility for regular checkups. During the examination, the client reveals that she is addicted to alcohol and tobacco. The client is concerned; she wants to provide a healthy environment for her unborn child and also know how to avoid harmful consequences.

1. What is the role of the nurse in handling substance-abusing mothers?

_____

_____

_____

2. How can the nurse use the "5 A's" approach to help this client attempt to quit smoking?

_____

_____

_____

SECTION IV: PRACTICING FOR NCLEX

Activity F *Answer the following questions.*

1. A newborn at a health care facility requires resuscitation. Which of the following condi-

tions should a nurse assess for to determine an increased risk of meconium aspiration syndrome in a newborn?

a. High-pitched cry

b. Bile-stained emesis

c. Increased intracranial pressure

d. End-expiratory grunting

2. A newborn in a family maternity center is suspected of having a cardiopulmonary disorder. Which of the following symptoms of persistent pulmonary hypertension should the nurse assess for in the newborn?

a. Systolic ejection murmur

b. Respiratory alkalosis

c. Rhinorrhea

d. Lacrimation

3. A nurse is caring for an infant born after a prolonged and difficult maternal labor. What are the nursing interventions involved when assessing for trauma and birth injuries in the newborn?

a. Examine the newborn's skin for cyanosis

b. Be alert for signs of apathy and listlessness

c. Assess the baby for any temperature instability

d. Note any absence of or decrease in deep tendon reflexes

4. A nurse is assigned to care for a newborn with hyperbilirubinemia. The newborn is relatively large in size and shows signs of listlessness. The nurse understands that which of the following could have caused these conditions to occur in the infant?

a. The infant's mother must have had a low birth weight

b. The infant's mother must have been a diabetic

c. The infant must have experienced birth trauma

d. The infant's mother must have abused alcohol

5. A nurse is caring for a newborn with periventricular–intraventricular hemorrhage in a local health care facility. Which of the following complications are likely to occur in a newborn with periventricular–intraventricular hemorrhage that a nurse should assess for? Select all that apply.

a. Hydrocephalus

b. Acid–base imbalances

c. Pneumonitis

d. Vision or hearing deficits

e. Cerebral palsy

6. A nurse is caring for a newborn whose chest x-ray reveals marked hyperaeration mixed with areas of atelectasis. The infant's arterial blood gas analysis indicates metabolic acidosis. The nurse should prepare for the assessment of which of the following dangerous conditions when providing care to this newborn?

a. Choanal atresia

b. Necrotizing enterocolitis

c. Meconium aspiration syndrome

d. Hyperbilirubinemia

7. A nurse is caring for a newborn with transient tachypnea in a family maternity center. Which of the following is an important nursing intervention for a newborn with transient tachypnea?

a. Administer IV fluids; gavage feedings

b. Maintain adequate hydration

c. Monitor for signs of hypotonia

d. Perform gentle suctioning

8. A nurse in a local family maternity center is caring for a newborn with asphyxia. What nursing management is involved when treating a newborn with asphyxia?

a. Ensure adequate tissue perfusion

b. Ensure effective resuscitation measures

c. Administer intravenous (IV) fluids

d. Administer surfactant as ordered

9. A nurse is caring for a newborn with esophageal atresia that had occurred during early fetal development. What should the preoperative nursing care for the newborn focus on?

a. Document the amount and color of drainage

b. Administer antibiotics and total parenteral nutrition as ordered

c. Prevent aspiration by elevating the head of the bed

d. Provide colostomy care if required

10. A client has delivered a newborn in a local health care facility. The client has experienced substance abuse. Which of the following interventions should the nurse perform when caring for a newborn of this client?

a. Encourage early initiation of feedings

b. Monitor newborn's cardiovascular status

c. Supplement breast milk with formula

d. Check newborn's skin turgor and fontanels

11. A nurse is caring for a newborn with jaundice undergoing phototherapy. Which of the following interventions should the nurse perform when caring for the newborn?

a. Expose the newborn's skin minimally

b. Shield the newborn's eyes

c. Discourage feeding the newborn

d. Discontinue therapy if stools are loose, green, and frequent

12. A nurse is caring for a newborn with meconium aspiration syndrome. Which of the following interventions should the nurse perform when caring for this newborn? Select all that apply.

a. Perform repeated suctioning and stimulation

b. Place the newborn under a radiant warmer or in a warmed Isolette

c. Handle and rub the newborn well with a dry towel

d. Administer oxygen therapy

e. Administer broad-spectrum antibiotics

13. A newborn with feeding intolerance is suspected of having gastroschisis. Which of the following characteristics of gastroschisis should the nurse know when assessing the newborn?

a. No peritoneal sac protecting herniated organs

b. Normal herniated organs

c. It is a defect of the umbilical ring

d. Resolves with surgical correction

14. A nurse is caring for a newborn with necrotizing enterocolitis, scheduled to undergo surgery for bowel resection. The infant's parents wish to know the implications of the surgery. Which of the following information should the nurse provide the parents regarding surgery to treat necrotizing enterocolitis?

    a. Surgically treated NEC is a short process

    b. Surgery will prevent long-term medical problems

    c. Surgery requires placement of a proximal enterostomy

    d. Surgery prevents the use of long-term antibiotics

15. Bronchopulmonary dysplasia (BPD) is the result of lung injury in the newborn. What can be done to reduce the incidence of BPD in the newborn?

    a. Antepartal administration of steroids to the mother

    b. Mechanical ventilation of the newborn with 100% oxygen content

    c. Steroid injection at birth to all infants at risk for BPD

    d. Exogenous surfactant given to the mother prior to the baby's birth

16. Congenital heart anomalies affect approximately 8 infants in every 1,000 live births. The nursing assessment should include what important information that might indicate heart failure in the infant?

    a. Capillary refill time

    b. Diminished peripheral pulses

    c. Color of hands and feet

    d. Blood glucose level

17. Providing nursing care to a newborn born with a congenital cardiac anomaly can be a challenging task. What is a priority component of providing nursing care to the newborn with a congenital cardiac anomaly?

    a. Oversee laboratory procedures

    b. Accompany the newborn to all radiologic examinations

    c. Prevent pain as much as possible

    d. Teach the parents to take pulse and blood pressure measurements

18. Spina bifida is a general term used to denote the condition where there is a defect in the vertebral column. It can range from mild to severe, and its effects are specific to the region of the deformity. What is the more precise term used to describe a herniation through the skin of the back when both the spinal cord and nerve roots are involved?

    a. Meningocele

    b. Spina bifida occulta

    c. Spina bifida cystica

    d. Myelomeningocele

19. Infants born with spina bifida are at increased risk for hydrocephalus. What is the priority nursing assessment for an infant at risk for hydrocephalus?

    a. Assess the level of irritability

    b. Assess the weight

    c. Assess head circumference

    d. Assess movement of the lower extremities

20. Infants born with a diaphragmatic hernia are given supportive treatment until they can have surgery to repair the defect. What are the medications usually given to these infants? Select all that apply.

    a. Steroids

    b. Inotropics

    c. Surfactant

    d. Plasma expanders

    e. Bronchodilators

21. A newborn with a cleft lip and palate often provide challenges to the parents when providing care prior to surgical repair of the defects. At what age is the defect in the lip usually repaired?

    a. 2-6 weeks

    b. 6-12 weeks

    c. 2-3 months

    d. 6-12 months

22. A relatively common birth defect, hypospadias, occurs when the urethral meatus is found on the underside of the penis instead of at the tip. What is it often accompanied by that can lead to problems urinating?

    a. Chordee
    b. Prepuce
    c. Priapism
    d. Cholangi

23. Congenital club foot can take one of two forms, either rigid or supple. The type of congenital club foot dictates the treatment involved in its correction, even though the initial treatment for both types of club foot is the same. What is the initial treatment for an infant born with a congenital club foot?

    a. Surgery
    b. Braces
    c. Physical therapy
    d. Serial casting

24. Developmental dysplasia of the hip is often not identified at birth. A careful nursing assessment often identifies this problem in a newborn. What procedure does a nurse perform to get the sensation of the dislocated hip going back into the acetabulum?

    a. Ortolani's maneuver
    b. Barlow's maneuver
    c. Pavlik's maneuver
    d. Bill's maneuver

25. What are the causes of retinopathy of the preterm newborn? Select all that apply.

    a. Insufficient oxygenation in an Isolette
    b. Assistive ventilation with high oxygen content
    c. Acidosis
    d. Alkalosis
    e. Shock

Answers

CHAPTER 1

Activity A

1. doula
2. Intrauterine
3. breast
4. family
5. emancipated
6. specialty
7. discipline
8. competence
9. anticipatory
10. Morbidity

Activity B

1. d   **2.** e   **3.** b   **4.** c   **5.** a

Activity C

1.

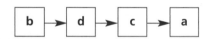

Activity D

1. Nurses need to take care and look beyond the obvious "crushing chest pain" symptom that heralds a heart attack in men because women present symptoms of CVD in a very different way, and the diagnosis is missed if CVD is not on their list of possibilities. Nurses should, therefore, monitor the following risk factors in women that could lead to CVD:
   - Cigarette smoking
   - Smoking and use of oral contraceptives or hormone replacement therapy
   - Obesity
   - A diet high in saturated fats
   - Stress
   - Sedentary lifestyle
   - Hypertension
   - Hyperlipidemia
   - Strong family history
   - Diabetes mellitus
   - Postmenopausal
2. Case management is a collaborative process involving assessment, planning, implementation, coordination, monitoring, and evaluation. It includes advocacy, communication, resource management, client-focused comprehensive care across a continuum, and coordinated care with an interdisciplinary approach.
3. Risk factors for breast cancer in women include the following:
   - Positive family history of breast cancer
   - Aging
   - Irregularities in the menstrual cycle at an early age
   - Excess weight
   - Not having children
   - Oral contraceptive use
   - Excessive alcohol consumption
   - A high-fat diet
   - Long-term use of hormone replacement therapy
4. Evidence-based nursing practice involves the use of research or evidence in establishing a plan of care and implementing that care. It is a problem-solving approach to nursing clinical decisions. This concept of nursing practice includes the use of the best current evidence in making decisions about the care of women, children, and their families.
5. Maternal mortality rate measures the number of deaths from any cause during the pregnancy cycle per 100,000 live births.
6. Low birth weight and prematurity are major indicators of infant health and significant predictors of infant mortality. The lower the birth weight, the higher the risk of infant mortality.

Activity E

1. Our hospital defines "family-centered care" as the delivery of safe, satisfying, high-quality health care that focuses on and adapts to the physical and psychosocial needs of the family. It is a cooperative effort of families and other caregivers that recognizes the strength and integrity of the family. What that really means is that when you come in to have your baby, we will not only take care of you and your newborn, we will also include your husband as part of your family unit. We will listen to what you and your husband want and include it in your plan of care as best we can.
2. "Evidence-based nursing practice" involves the use of research or evidence in establishing a plan of care

for you and your newborn and implementing that care. This model of nursing practice includes the use of the best current evidence in making decisions about care.

Activity F

1. Answer: b
RATIONALE: Breastfeeding reduces the rates of infection in infants and helps to improve long-term maternal health. Placing the infant on his or her back to sleep prevents sudden infant death syndrome (SIDS) but does not prevent infections in the infant. Feeding foods high in starch or feeding liquids frequently will not prevent infections either.

2. Answer: a
RATIONALE: The nurses should advocate adequate intake of folic acid supplements during pregnancy to reduce the prevalence of neural defects in infants. Taking vitamin E supplements, engaging in mild exercises during pregnancy, and regularly consuming citrus fruits are healthy habits for the mother and infant, but they do not reduce the risk of developing neural defects among infants.

3. Answer: d
RATIONALE: According to the ANA's code of ethics, the nurse could make arrangements for alternate care providers for a client undergoing an abortion, if the nurse ethically opposes the procedure. Nurses need to make their values and beliefs known to their managers before the situation occurs so that alternate staffing arrangement can be made. Under the ANA's code of ethics for nurses, the nurse need not provide emotional support to the client nor should he or she involve the client's family in convincing the client against an abortion.

4. Answer: d
RATIONALE: The nurse should instruct the client to place her infant on his or her back to sleep to prevent SIDS. Draping the infant in warm clothes, providing very soft bedding, or feeding a mixture of salts, sugar, and water will not prevent SIDS in the infant.

5. Answer: b
RATIONALE: Lung cancer has no early symptoms, making its early detection almost impossible. Lung cancer is equally fatal for both men and women; it is not more deadly in men. Women do not have a stronger resistance to lung cancer. It is the most common cancer in women due to the increasing frequency of smoking. Although the early detection of lung cancer is very difficult, its diagnosis is not more challenging in women than in men.

6. Answer: c
RATIONALE: A traditional method used in this country to measure health is to examine mortality and morbidity data. Information is collected and analyzed to provide an objective description of the nation's health. Tracking the incidence of violent crime does not give information on the health

status of this country; neither does examining health disparities between ethnic groups or identifying specific national goals related to maternal and infant care without acting on the information.

7. Answer: c
RATIONALE: In the Arab-American culture, women are subordinate to men. The nurse would deal directly and exclusively with the husband. This family would not place much emphasis on preventive care either. Inquiring about folk remedies used may be appropriate with African-American families. Coordinating care through the client's mother might be appropriate with a Hispanic family.

8. Answer: b
RATIONALE: Clients have the right to refuse medical treatment, based on the American Hospital Association's Bill of Rights. The nurse needs to heed the client's wishes and not give the medication.

9. Answer: d
RATIONALE: The nurse should tell the client that the law specifically states that it is her decision who can see her health records and who cannot.

10. Answer: c
RATIONALE: In cases of abuse and violence, nurses can serve their clients best by not trying to rescue them but by helping them build on their strengths, providing support, and empowering them to help themselves. Counseling the client's partner against abuse, helping her know the legal impact of her situation, and introducing the client to a women's rights group to garner support are not the best ways of serving the client.

CHAPTER 2

Activity A

1. Nonverbal
2. Case
3. Community
4. Outpatient
5. prevention
6. family-centered
7. competence
8. encounters
9. Health
10. fragile

Activity B

1. The figure depicts the three levels of prevention in community-based nursing. At the primary level, the nurse provides anticipatory guidance and family teaching. Secondary prevention is the early detection and treatment of adverse health conditions. Tertiary prevention is designed to reduce or limit the progression of a disease or disability after an injury.

Activity C

1. d   **2.** c   **3.** b   **4.** a

Activity D

1.

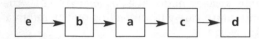

Activity E

1. Some of the techniques that the nurse can use to enhance learning include:
   - Slowing down and repeating information often
   - Speaking in conversational style using plain, non-medical language
   - "Chunking" information and teaching it in small bites using logical steps
   - Prioritizing information and teaching "survival skills" first
   - Using visuals, such as pictures, videos, and models
   - Teaching using an interactive, "hands-on" approach

2. The four main purposes of nursing documentation are:
   - The client's medical record serves as a communication tool that the entire interdisciplinary team can use to keep track of what the client and family has learned already and what learning still needs to occur.
   - It serves to testify to the education the family has received if and when legal matters arise.
   - It verifies standards set by the JCAHO, Centers for Medicare and Medicaid Services (CMS), and other accrediting bodies that hold health care providers accountable for client education activities.
   - It informs third-party payers of goods and services provided for reimbursement purposes.

3. The nurse in an outpatient clinic will provide
   - Health screening
   - Education
   - Medication administration
   - Telephone consultation
   - Health system referral
   - Instruction
   - Nutritional counseling
   - Risk identification

4. Both contribute to improved transition from the hospital to the community for women, their families, and the health care team.

5. During the past several years, the health care delivery system has changed dramatically. With a focus on cost containment, people are spending less time in the hospital. Patients are being discharged "sicker and quicker" from their hospital beds. The health care system has moved from reactive treatment strategies in hospitals to a proactive approach in the community. This has resulted in an increasing emphasis on health promotion and illness prevention within the community.

6. A birthing center provides a cross between a home birth and a hospital birth. Birthing centers offer a homelike setting with close proximity to a hospital in case of complications. Midwives often are the sole care providers in freestanding birthing centers, with obstetricians as backups in case of emergencies. Birthing centers usually have fewer restrictions and guidelines for families to follow and allow for more freedom in making laboring decisions. Birthing centers aim to provide a relaxing home environment and promote a culture of normalcy.

Activity F

1. The nurse should adapt to different cultural beliefs and practices by:
   - Being flexible and accepting of others' points of view
   - Listening to clients and learning about their beliefs about health and wellness
   - Knowing, understanding, and respecting culturally influenced health behaviors

2. Some of the cultural characteristics that would be important for a nurse to understand include:
   - Values
   - Beliefs of the various people to whom they deliver care
   - Time orientation
   - Personal space
   - Language
   - Family orientation

3. To ensure culturally competent nursing care to diverse families, the nurse should:
   - Develop cultural self-awareness
   - Gain cultural knowledge about various world views of different cultures
   - Participate in cultural encounters

Activity G

1. **Answer: d**
   RATIONALE: Case management focuses on coordinating health care services while balancing quality and cost outcomes. Helping a family member learn how to perform a procedure is part of the teaching role. Assessing sanitary conditions is done during discharge planning, and establishing eligibility for Medicaid is resource management.

2. **Answer: a**
   RATIONALE: Key elements in the provision of family-centered care include demonstrating interpersonal sensitivity, providing general health information and being a valuable resource, communicating specific health information, and treating people respectfully (Mullen, Conrad, Hoadley, & Iannone, 2007). Giving as much control as possible to the client and their family is essential in family-centered care. Give all the health information, both good and bad, that the client or their family request. Be culturally sensitive to your client and their family.

3. **Answer: c**
   RATIONALE: Asking questions or having private conversations with the interpreter may make the family uncomfortable and destroy the patient–nurse

relationship. Translation takes longer than a same-language appointment, and this must be considered so that the family is not rushed. A nonprofessional may be unable to adequately translate medical terminology. Using a relative can upset the family relationships or cause legal problems.

4. **Answer: a**
RATIONALE: Recognizing family strengths and individuality is a key element of family-centered home care. Ensuring a safe, nurturing environment is part of the assessment process prior to preparing the nursing plan of care. Information should be shared completely and openly with parents, not "managed." The nurse should respect different methods of coping rather than correcting them.

5. **Answer: b**
RATIONALE: Promoting the health and safety of a group of clients is a common goal of nurses in all community settings. Removing health barriers to learning is the community nurse's goal. Determining the type of care a client needs is the goal of telephone triage. Ensuring the health and well-being of women and their families is a goal of family-centered home care.

6. **Answer: b**
RATIONALE: The nurse should monitor for the incidence of hydrocephalus in the high-risk newborn. Hydrocephalus, along with conditions such as cerebral palsy, retinopathy, and ongoing oxygen dependency, is likely to persist after discharge in a high-risk newborn. Anencephaly and fetal distress syndrome are not conditions that persist after discharge. Spina bifida is most often noted at birth and would not to need to be assessed for by the nurse.

7. **Answer: b**
RATIONALE: The nurse should instruct the client to take folic acid supplements, as consumption of folic acid supplements reduces the risk of developing NTDs in the growing fetus. Taking vitamin E supplements and consuming legumes and citrus fruits regularly during pregnancy do not reduce the risk of developing NTDs.

8. **Answer: d**
RATIONALE: The nurse should inform the women that comprehensive community-centered care should be given to women during their reproductive years. This is because as their reproductive goals change, so do their health care needs. A women's immune system does not weaken immediately after birth. Similarly, women do not have more health problems specifically during their reproductive years, nor are they more susceptible to stress during their reproductive years.

9. **Answer: b**
RATIONALE: The nurse should include the monitoring of the physical and emotional well-being of the client's family members as part of her postpartum care in the home environment. The nurse should provide hands-on experience in infant care instead of providing self-help books to the client. The nurse should include parental needs along with the infant needs and focus on each of its areas while preparing her discharge plan, as the nurse should identify potential or developing complications not only in the infant but also in the client.

10. **Answer: a**
RATIONALE: A nurse who thinks stereotypically may assign a client to a staff member who is of the same culture as the client because the nurse assumes that all people of that culture are alike. The nurse also may believe that clients with the same skin color may react in the same manner in similar social situations. Because stereotypes are preconceived ideas unsupported by facts, they may not be real or accurate. In fact, they can be dangerous because they are dehumanizing and interfere with accepting others as unique individuals.

CHAPTER 3

Activity A
1. rugae
2. Prolactin
3. epididymis
4. urethra
5. endometrium
6. Skene's
7. episiotomy
8. prostate
9. uterus
10. scrotum

Activity B

1. a. The figure shows the lateral view of the internal
female reproductive organs.

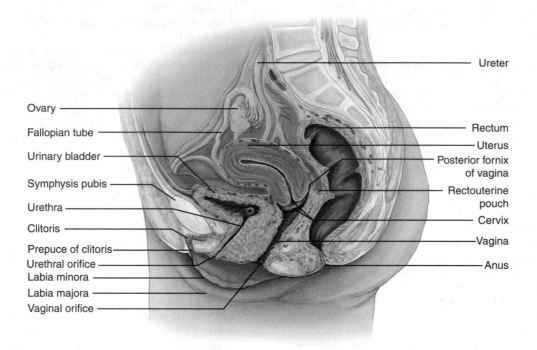

Ovary

Fallopian tube

Urinary bladder

Symphysis pubis

Urethra

Clitoris

Prepuce of clitoris

Urethral orifice

Labia minora

Labia majora

Vaginal orifice

Ureter

Rectum

Uterus

Posterior fornix
of vagina

Rectouterine
pouch

Cervix

Vagina

Anus

b. The internal female reproductive organs consist
of the vagina, uterus, fallopian tubes, and ovaries.
The vagina is a canal that connects the external
genitals to the uterus. It receives the penis and the
sperm ejaculated during sexual intercourse, and it
serves as an exit passageway for menstrual blood
and for the fetus during childbirth. The uterus is a
pear-shaped muscular organ at the top of the
vagina. It is the site of menstruation, implantation of a fertilized ovum, development of the
fetus during pregnancy, and labor. The fallopian
tubes are hollow, cylindrical structures that ex-
tend 2 to 3 inches from the upper edges of the
uterus toward the ovaries. The fallopian tubes
convey the ovum from the ovary to the uterus
and sperm from the uterus toward the ovary. The
ovaries are a set of paired glands resembling un-
shelled almonds set in the pelvic cavity below
and to either side of the umbilicus. The development and release of the ovum and the secretion
of the hormones estrogen and progesterone are
the two primary functions of the ovary.

2. a. The figure shows the lateral view of the internal male reproductive organs.

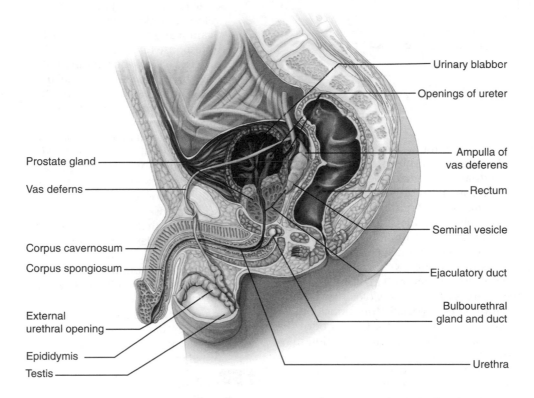

- Urinary bladder
- Openings of ureter
- Ampulla of vas deferens
- Rectum
- Seminal vesicle
- Ejaculatory duct
- Bulbourethral gland and duct
- Urethra

Prostate gland
Vas deferns
Corpus cavernosum
Corpus spongiosum
External urethral opening
Epididymis
Testis

b. The internal structures include the testes, the ductal system, and accessory glands. The testes are oval bodies the size of large olives that lie in the scrotum. They produce sperm and synthesize testosterone. The vas deferens is a cordlike duct that transports sperm from the epididymis. The seminal vesicles, which produce nutrient seminal fluid, and the prostate gland, which produces alkaline prostatic fluid, are both connected to the ejaculatory duct leading into the urethra. The bulbourethral glands secrete a mucus-like fluid in response to sexual stimulation and lubricate the head of the penis in preparation for sexual intercourse.

3. The figure shows the internal structures of a testis.

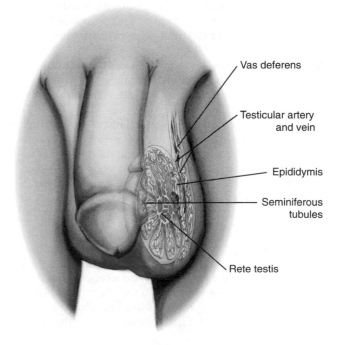

- Vas deferens
- Testicular artery and vein
- Epididymis
- Seminiferous tubules
- Rete testis

Activity C

1. e   2. c   3. b   4. d   5. a

Activity D

1.

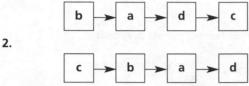

2.

Activity E

1. The external female reproductive organs collectively are called the vulva. The vulva serves to protect the urethral and vaginal openings. The structures that make up the vulva include the mons pubis, the labia majora and minora, the clitoris, the structures within the vestibule, and the perineum.

2. Soon after childbirth, colostrum is secreted for approximately a week, with gradual conversion to mature milk. Colostrum is a dark yellow fluid that contains more minerals and protein, but less sugar and fat, than mature breast milk. Colostrum is rich in maternal antibodies, especially immunoglobulin A (IgA), which offers protection for the newborn against enteric pathogens. Colostrum secretion may continue after childbirth.

3. During the perimenopausal years, women may experience physical changes associated with decreasing estrogen levels, which may include vasomotor symptoms of hot flashes, irregular menstrual cycles, sleep disruptions, forgetfulness, irritability, mood disturbances, decreased vaginal lubrication, fatigue, vaginal atrophy, and depression.

4. Nurses can play a major role in assisting menopausal women by educating and counseling them about the multitude of options available for disease prevention, treatment for menopausal symptoms, and health promotion during this time of change in their lives.

5. The testes produce sperm and synthesize testosterone, which is the primary male sex hormone. Sperm is produced in the seminiferous tubules of the testes.

6. The bulbourethral (Cowper's) glands are two small structures about the size of peas, located inferior to the prostate gland. They are composed of several tubes whose epithelial linings secrete a mucus-like fluid. It is released in response to sexual stimulation and lubricates the head of the penis in preparation for sexual intercourse. They gradually diminish in size with advancing age.

Activity F

1. a. The nurse should inform Susan about the following: the main function of the reproductive cycle is to stimulate growth of a follicle to release an egg and prepare a site for implantation if fertilization occurs; menstruation, the monthly shedding of the uterine lining, marks the beginning of a new cycle; the menstrual cycle involves a complex interaction of hormones; the ovarian cycle is the series of events associated with a developing oocyte (ovum, or egg) within the ovaries; at ovulation, a mature follicle ruptures in response to a surge of LH, releasing a mature oocyte (ovum); the endometrial cycle is divided into three phases: the follicular or proliferative phase, the luteal or secretory phase, and the menstrual phase; the endometrium, ovaries, pituitary gland, and hypothalamus are all involved in the cyclic changes that help to prepare the body for fertilization; the menstrual cycle results from a functional hypothalamic-pituitary-ovarian axis and a precise sequencing of hormones that lead to ovulation; if conception doesn't occur, menses ensues; and the one thing to remember is that whether a women's cycle is 28 days or 120 days, ovulation takes place 14 days before menstruation.

   b. The nurse should inform Susan that cycles vary in frequency from 21 to 36 days; bleeding lasts 3 to 8 days; blood loss averages 20 to 80 mL; the average cycle is 28 days long, but this varies; and irregular menses can be associated with irregular ovulation, stress, disease, and hormonal imbalances.

Activity G

1. **Answer: b**
   RATIONALE: To increase the chances of conceiving, the best time for intercourse is one or two days before ovulation. This ensures that the sperm meets the ovum at the right time. The average life of a sperm cell is two to three days, and the sperm cells will not be able to survive until ovulation if intercourse occurs a week before ovulation. The chances of conception are minimal for intercourse after ovulation.

2. **Answer: d**
   RATIONALE: Bartholin's glands, when stimulated, secrete mucus that supplies lubrication for intercourse. Endocrine glands secrete hormones for various bodily functions. The pituitary gland releases follicle-stimulating hormone (FSH) to stimulate the ovary to produce follicles. Skene's glands secrete a small amount of mucus to keep the opening to the urethra moist and lubricated for the passage of urine.

3. **Answer: a**
   RATIONALE: The endometrium is the mucosal layer that lines the uterine cavity in nonpregnant women. The fundus is the convex portion above the uterine tubes. The mons pubis is the elevated, rounded, fleshy prominence over the symphysis pubis. The clitoris is a small, cylindrical mass of erectile tissue and nerves located at the anterior junction of the labia minora.

4. **Answer: b**

   RATIONALE: The nurse should inform the client that the yellow fluid is called colostrum, and it contains more minerals and protein, but less sugar and fat, than mature breast milk and is also rich in maternal antibodies. The nurse should inform the client that, gradually, the production of colostrum stops and the production of regular breast milk begins, but there is no need to avoid breastfeeding when colostrum is being produced, if the client's culture allows for it. There is no need to modify diet or to feed formula to the infant.

5. **Answer: c**

   RATIONALE: During ovulation, some women can feel a pain around the time the egg is released on one side of the abdomen. The pain is not a sign of pregnancy, as the client experiences this pain regularly during ovulation. The pain is also not related to an irregular menstruation cycle or the client's exercise regimen.

6. **Answer: b**

   RATIONALE: The nurse should inform the client that there will be a significant increase in temperature, usually 0.5 to 1° F, within a day or two after ovulation has occurred. The temperature remains elevated for 12 to 16 days, until menstruation begins. During ovulation, some women can feel a pain on one side of the abdomen around the time the egg is released. There is no significant correlation between ovulation and lack of sleep or feeling uneasiness or sickness.

7. **Answer: b**

   RATIONALE: After menopause, the uterus shrinks and gradually atrophies. A full bladder, not menopause, causes the uterus to tilt backward. Cervical muscle content does not increase during menopause. Menopause has no significant effect on the outer layer of the cervix.

8. **Answer: d**

   RATIONALE: Progesterone is called the hormone of pregnancy because it reduces uterine contractions, thus producing a calming effect on the uterus, allowing pregnancy to be maintained. Follicle-stimulating hormone (FSH) is primarily responsible for the maturation of the ovarian follicle. Luteinizing hormone (LH) is required for both the final maturation of preovulatory follicles and luteinization of the ruptured follicle. Estrogen is crucial for the development and maturation of the follicle.

9. **Answer: c**

   RATIONALE: During cold conditions, the scrotum is pulled closer to the body for warmth or protection. The cremaster muscles in the scrotal wall contract to allow the testes to be pulled closer to the body. Frequency of urination has no significant impact in maintaining the scrotal temperature. Increase in blood flow to the genital area occurs primarily during erection and is not due to climatic conditions.

10. **Answer: a**

    RATIONALE: With age, the prostate gland gradually enlarges, leading to difficulty during urination. Production of semen never stops, even though the quantity of semen produced may decrease. The prostate gland is not associated with painful erection. During the normal aging process, the prostate gland does not stop functioning, even though its capacity may be somewhat diminished.

11. **Answer: b**

    RATIONALE: The epididymis provides the space and environment for sperm to mature. The testes produce sperm, but they have to mature in the epididymis to become capable of impregnating the ovum. The vas deferens is the organ that transports sperm from the epididymis. The Cowper's glands secrete mucus-like fluid for lubrication during sexual intercourse.

12. **Answer: c**

    RATIONALE: The nurse should inform the client that the duration of the flow is about 3 to 7 days. An average cycle length is about 21 to 36 days, not 15 to 20 days. In the ovary, 2 million oocytes are present at birth, and about 400,000 follicles are still present at puberty. Blood loss averages 20 to 80 mL, not 120 to 150 mL.

13. **Answer: c**

    RATIONALE: At ovulation, a mature follicle ruptures, releasing a mature oocyte (ovum). Ovulation always takes place 14 days, not 10 days, before menstruation. The lifespan of the ovum is only about 24 hours, not 48 hours; unless it meets a sperm on its journey within that time, it will die. When ovulation occurs, there is a drop, not a rise, in estrogen levels.

14. **Answer: b**

    RATIONALE: Gonadotropin-releasing hormone is secreted from the hypothalamus in a pulsatile manner throughout the reproductive cycle. It induces the release of follicle-stimulating hormone and luteinizing hormone to assist with ovulation, both of which are secreted by the anterior pituitary gland. Estrogen is secreted by the ovaries and is crucial for the development and maturation of the follicle.

CHAPTER 4

Activity A

1. Adenomyosis
2. prostaglandin
3. Laparoscopy
4. perimenopause
5. vasectomy
6. medical
7. Osteoporosis
8. spinnbarkeit
9. basal
10. minipills

Activity B

1. This is a diaphragm. A diaphragm is used in conjunction with a spermicidal jelly or cream and inserted into the vagina to prevent the sperm from reaching the ovum.
2. **a.** The vas deferens is being cut with surgical scissors during a vasectomy.
   b. After a vasectomy, the semen no longer contains sperm, because the vas deferens (which carries sperm from the testes to the penis) is surgically cut.

Activity C

1. c　　**2.** d　　**3.** a　　**4.** e　　**5.** b

Activity D

1.

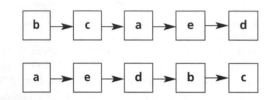

2.

Activity E

1. Common laboratory tests ordered to determine the cause of amenorrhea are karyotype, ultrasound to detect ovarian cysts, pregnancy test, thyroid function studies, prolactin level, follicle-stimulating hormone level, luteinizing hormone level, 17-ketosteroids tests, laparoscopy, and CT scan of head.
2. Menopause refers to the cessation of regular menstrual cycles. It is the end of menstruation and childbearing capacity. Natural menopause is defined as one year without a menstrual period. The average age at which it occurs is 51 years.
3. The risk factors associated with endometriosis are increasing age, family history of endometriosis, short menstrual cycle, long menstrual flow, young age at menarche, and few or no pregnancies.
4. Infertility is defined as the inability to conceive a child after one year of regular sexual intercourse unprotected by contraception, or the inability to carry a pregnancy to term.
5. In the Two-Day Method, women observe the presence or absence of cervical secretions by examining toilet paper or underwear or by monitoring their physical sensations. Every day, the woman asks two simple questions: "Did I note any secretions yesterday?" and "Did I note any secretions today?" If the answer to either question is yes, she considers herself fertile and avoids unprotected intercourse. If the answers are no, she is unlikely to become pregnant from unprotected intercourse on that day.
6. Intrauterine systems (IUSs) are small, plastic, T-shaped objects that are placed inside the uterus to provide contraception. They prevent pregnancy by making the endometrium of the uterus hostile to implantation of a fertilized ovum, by causing a nonspecific inflammatory reaction.

Activity F

1. Amenorrhea is a normal feature in prepubertal, pregnant, and postmenopausal women. The two categories of amenorrhea are primary and secondary amenorrhea. Primary amenorrhea is defined as either (1) absence of menses by age 14, with absence of growth and development of secondary sexual characteristics, or (2) absence of menses by age 16, with normal development of secondary sexual characteristics. Ninety-eight percent of American girls menstruate by age 16.
2. Causes of primary amenorrhea related to Alexa may include extreme weight gain or loss, stress from a major life event, excessive exercise, or eating disorders such as anorexia nervosa or bulimia. Primary amenorrhea is also caused by congenital abnormalities of the reproductive system, Cushing's disease, polycystic ovarian syndrome, hypothyroidism, and Turner syndrome; other causes are imperforate hymen, chronic illness, pregnancy, cystic fibrosis, congenital heart disease, and ovarian or adrenal tumors.
3. The treatment of primary amenorrhea involves correcting any underlying disorders as well as providing estrogen replacement therapy to stimulate the development of secondary sexual characteristics. If a pituitary tumor is the cause, it might be treated with drug therapy, surgical resection, or radiation therapy. Surgery might be needed to correct any structural abnormalities of the genital tract.
4. The nurse should address the diverse causes of amenorrhea, the relationship to sexual identity, and the possibility of infertility and more serious problems. In addition, the nurse should inform Alexa about the purpose of each diagnostic test, how it is performed, and when the results will be available. Sensitive listening, interviewing, and presenting treatment options are paramount to gaining the client's cooperation and understanding. Nutritional counseling is also vital in managing this disorder, especially when the client has findings suggestive of an eating disorder. Although not all causes can be addressed by making lifestyle changes, the nurse can still emphasize maintaining a healthy lifestyle.

Activity G

1. **Answer: d**
   RATIONALE: When assessing a client for amenorrhea, the nurse should document facial hair and acne as possible evidence of androgen excess secondary to a tumor. The nurse may observe and should document hypothermia, bradycardia, hypotension, and reduced subcutaneous fat in women with anorexia nervosa; however, these are not symptoms of excess androgen.

2. Answer: b

RATIONALE: The nurse should explain to the client that the fertility awareness method relies on the assumption that the "unsafe period" is approximately 6 days; 3 days before and 3 days after ovulation. The method also assumes that sperm can live up to 5 days, not just 24 hours after intercourse. An ovum lives up to 24 hours after being released from the ovary. The exact time of ovulation cannot be determined, so two to three days are added to the beginning and end to avoid pregnancy.

3. Answer: b, d, & e

RATIONALE: When instructing a client with dysmenorrhea on how to manage her symptoms, the nurse should ask her to increase water consumption, use heating pads or take warm baths, and increase exercise and physical activity. Water consumption serves as a natural diuretic; heating pads or warm baths help increase comfort; and exercise increases endorphins and suppresses prostaglandin release. The nurse should also tell the client to limit salty foods to prevent fluid retention during menstruation and to keep legs elevated while lying down, because this helps increase comfort.

4. Answer: d

RATIONALE: The nurse should prepare the client for a laparoscopy to obtain a definitive diagnosis; laparoscopy allows for direct visualization of the internal organs and helps confirm the diagnosis. A hysterosalpingogram (HSG) assesses tubal patency, and a clomiphene citrate challenge test determines ovarian function; these tests are not used to determine the extent of endometriosis.

5. Answer: d

RATIONALE: The nurse should instruct the client to deliver the semen sample to the laboratory for analysis within 1 to 2 hours after ejaculation. The client should also be instructed to collect the sample in a specimen container, not a condom or plastic bag. The client needs to abstain from sexual activity for at least 24 hours before giving the sample, but he need not avoid strenuous activity.

6. Answer: c

RATIONALE: The nurse should explain that during ovulation the cervix is high or deep in the vagina. The os is slightly open during ovulation. Under the influence of estrogen during ovulation, the cervical mucus is copious and slippery and can be stretched between two fingers without breaking. It becomes thick and dry after ovulation, under the influence of progesterone.

7. Answer: c

RATIONALE: If the FSH level is greater than 15, the test is considered abnormal and the likelihood of conception with the client's own eggs is very low. Therefore, the nurse could suggest the use of donor eggs or gamete intrafallopian transfer as an option. Artificial insemination will not help solve the couple's problem. Also, it would be incorrect for the nurse to imply that the couple has no choice other than adoption.

8. Answer: c

RATIONALE: Recent studies have shown that the extended use of active OC pills carries the same safety profile as the conventional 28-day regimen. This option helps reduce the number of periods and is as effective as the conventional regimen. There is no evidence to suggest that discontinuation of active oral contraceptives will not ensure restoration of fertility. Depo-Provera, not active oral contraceptive pills, prevents pregnancy for three months at a time.

9. Answer: d

RATIONALE: The client should be instructed to take her temperature before rising and record it on a chart. If using this method by itself, the client should avoid unprotected intercourse until the BBT has been elevated for three days. The client should be informed that other fertility awareness methods should be used along with BBT for better results. The oral method is better suited than the axillary method for taking the temperature in this case.

10. Answer: d

RATIONALE: The best option for a client who is not well-educated would be the Standard Days Method with CycleBeads, since the 32 color-coded CycleBeads are easy to use and understand. An injection of Depo-Provera would also suit this client, since it works by suppressing ovulation and the production of FSH and LH by the pituitary gland and prevents pregnancy for 3 months at a time. Basal body temperature requires the client to take and chart her body temperature; this may be difficult for the client to follow. Coitus interruptus is a method in which the man controls his ejaculation and ejaculates outside the vagina; this suggests that the client rely solely on the cooperation and judgment of her spouse. The lactational amenorrhea method (LAM) works as a temporary method of contraception only for breastfeeding mothers.

11. Answer: a, c, & e

RATIONALE: The nurse should tell the client to inspect the cervical cap prior to insertion for cracks, holes, or tears and to wait approximately 30 minutes after insertion before engaging in sexual intercourse to be sure that a seal has formed between the rim and the cervix. In addition, the cap should not be used during menses because of the potential for toxic shock syndrome; an alternative method such as condoms should be used during this time. The client should be told not to apply spermicide to the rim since it may interfere with the seal. It should be left in place for a minimum of 6 hours after sexual intercourse.

12. Answer: b

RATIONALE: Because of the client's smoking habit, combination oral contraceptives may be contraindicated. Oral contraceptives are highly effective when taken properly but can aggravate many medical conditions, especially in women who smoke. The Lunelle injection, Depo-Provera, or copper intrauterine devices are not contraindicated in this client and can be used with certain precautions. Implantable contraceptives are subdermal time-release implants that deliver synthetic progestin; these are highly effective and are not contraindicated in this client.

13. **Answer: b**

RATIONALE: The client is seeking a medical abortion. The nurse should inform the client that such medications are effectively used to terminate a pregnancy only during the first trimester, not the second. The medications are available as a vaginal suppository or in oral form and do not present a high risk of respiratory failure. Sterilization, not abortion, is considered a permanent end to fertility.

14. **Answer: b**

RATIONALE: Since the client has multiple sex partners, condoms will help offer protection against sexually transmitted infections (STIs) and are best suited for her needs. The client cannot use an IUD because of her history of various pelvic infections. Although oral contraceptives (OCs) will help the client as a means of contraception, this method is not the best choice for her because it does not offer protection against STIs. Tubal ligation is a sterilization procedure and does not suit the client's purpose.

15 **Answer: b, c, & e**

RATIONALE: The nurse needs to clear up misconceptions by explaining to clients that taking birth control pills does not protect against STIs and that irregular menstruation or douching after sex does not prevent pregnancy. The nurse also needs to confirm that breastfeeding does not protect against pregnancy and that pregnancy can occur during menses.

16. **Answer: a**

RATIONALE: Since the client has a history of cardiac problems, long-term hormone replacement therapy (HRT) is contraindicated. This is because there is an increased risk of heart attacks and strokes. The client should instead be asked to consider options with minimized risk, such as lipid-lowering agents, or nonhormonal therapies, such as bisphosphonates and selective estrogen receptor modulators (SERMs).

17. **Answer: c**

RATIONALE: The client is likely to be experiencing vaginal atrophy, which occurs during menopause because of declining estrogen levels. The condition can be managed with the use of over-the-counter moisturizers and lubricants. A positive outlook on sexuality and a supportive partner may make the sexual experience enjoyable and fulfilling, while a support group may reduce the client's anxiety. However, these will not alleviate the client's discomfort. Menopause can be a physically and emotionally challenging time for women because of the stigma of an "aging" body;

the nurse should be sensitive to the client's feelings when discussing these changes.

18. **Answer: a**

RATIONALE: It is important for the nurse to initiate the treatment process by outlining the risks and benefits of treatments to couples with infertility; this helps the couple make an informed decision in a nondirective, nonjudgmental environment. The couple also should be made aware of the treatment options available and accessible to them. Based on the couple's financial status, the nurse should assist them in making a priority list of diagnostic tests and potential treatment options; this will help the couple plan their financial strategy. The couple's emotional distress is usually very high, so the nurse must be able to recognize that anxiety and provide emotional support during treatment.

19. **Answer: a**

RATIONALE: The nurse should inform the client that intrauterine systems cause monthly periods to become lighter, shorter, and less painful. Monthly periods reduce in number with use of oral contraceptives but not with use of intrauterine systems.

20. **Answer: b, c, & d**

RATIONALE: The nurse should instruct the client to wet the sponge before inserting it, to insert it 24 hours before intercourse, and to leave it in place for at least six hours following intercourse, to be effective. The sponge should not be replaced every two hours because this will reduce its efficacy. A contraceptive sponge covers the cervix and releases spermicide. It does not protect against STIs. Therefore, keeping the sponge for more than 30 hours will not prevent STIs but will increase risk of toxic shock syndrome.

CHAPTER 5

Activity A

1. Trichomoniasis
2. tertiary
3. Ectoparasites
4. Scabies
5. thrush
6. Syphilis
7. liver
8. chlamydia
9. CD4
10. chlamydia

Activity B

1. a. The disease is a sexually transmitted infection known as gonorrhea.
   b. If gonorrhea remains untreated, it can enter the bloodstream and produce a disseminated gonococcal infection. This severe form of infection can invade the joints (arthritis), the heart (endocarditis), the brain (meningitis), and the liver (toxic hepatitis).

2. **a.** The disease is a sexually transmitted infection known as trichomoniasis.
   b. The clinical manifestations of trichomoniasis include a heavy yellow/green or gray frothy or bubbly discharge, vaginal pruritus and vulvar soreness, dyspareunia, bleeding of cervix, dysuria, and colpitis macularis ("strawberry" look on cervix).

3. **a.** This is a sexually transmitted infection known as pelvic inflammatory disease.
   b. Pelvic inflammatory disease results from an ascending polymicrobial infection of the upper female reproductive tract, frequently caused by untreated chlamydia or gonorrhea.

Activity C

1. c   2. a   3. b   4. f   5. d
6. e

Activity D

1.

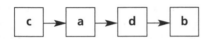

Activity E

1. Predisposing factors that may increase the chances of vulvovaginal candidiasis include pregnancy; use of oral contraceptives with a high estrogen content; use of broad-spectrum antibiotics; diabetes mellitus; use of steroids and immunosuppressive drugs; HIV infection; wearing tight, restrictive clothes and nylon underpants; and trauma to vaginal mucosa from chemical irritants or douching

2. Hepatitis A produces flulike symptoms with malaise, fatigue, anorexia, nausea, pruritus, fever, and upper-right-quadrant pain.

3. HIV is transmitted by intimate sexual contact; by sharing needles for intravenous drug use; from mother to fetus during pregnancy; or by transfusion of blood or blood products.

4. Acquired immunodeficiency syndrome (AIDS) is a breakdown in the immune function caused by HIV, a retrovirus. The infected person develops opportunistic infections or malignancies that become fatal. Progression from HIV infection to AIDS occurs at a median of 11 years after infection.

5. There can be hundreds of causes of vaginitis, but more often than not the cause is infection by one of three organisms: *Candida*, a fungus; *Trichomonas*, a protozoan; or *Gardnerella*, a bacterium.

6. The clinical manifestations of chlamydia are mucopurulent vaginal discharge, urethritis, bartholinitis, endometritis, salpingitis, and dysfunctional uterine bleeding.

Activity F

1. **a.** In pregnant women, gonorrhea is associated with chorioamnionitis, premature labor, premature rupture of membranes, and postpartum endometritis. It can also be transmitted to the newborn in the form of ophthalmia neonatorum during birth, by direct contact with gonococcal organisms in the cervix. Ophthalmia neonatorum is highly contagious and, if untreated, leads to blindness of the newborn.
   b. The nurse should be aware of the following factors:
   • Sensitivity and confidentiality: there is a social stigma attached to STIs, so women need to be reassured about confidentiality.
   • Education and counseling skills: the nurse should possess the necessary education and counseling skills to help the client deal with the infection.
   • Level of knowledge: the nurse's level of knowledge about chlamydia and gonorrhea should include treatment strategies, referral sources, and preventive measures.
   • Assessment: Assessment involves taking a health history that includes a comprehensive sexual history. Questions about the number of sex partners and the use of safer sex practices are appropriate. Previous and current symptoms should be reviewed. Seeking treatment and informing sex partners should be emphasized.
   c. High-risk groups who may develop gonorrhea include individuals who
   • Have low socioeconomic status
   • Live in an urban area
   • Are single
   • Practice inconsistent use of barrier contraceptives
   • Have multiple sex partners

Activity G

1. **Answer: c**
   RATIONALE: As a preventive measure for the client with frequent vulvovaginal candidiasis, the nurse should instruct the client to wear white, 100% cotton underpants. The nurse should instruct the client to use pads instead of superabsorbent tampons, to avoid douching the affected area (it washes away protective vaginal mucus), and to reduce her dietary intake of simple sugars and soda.

2. **Answer: a**
   RATIONALE: The nurse should instruct the client to use high-protein supplements such as Boost to provide quick and easy protein and calories. The nurse should also instruct the client to eat dry crackers upon arising, not after every meal, and to eat six small meals a day, not three. Drinking fluids constantly, while eating, is not recommended. The nurse should instruct the client to separate the intake of food and fluids.

3. **Answer: b**
   RATIONALE: The nurse should inform the client that even after warts are removed, HPV still remains and viral shedding will continue. The nurse should instruct the client to avoid applying steroid

creams, sprays, or gels to vaginal area. All women above the age of 30 should undergo an HPV test, and women between 9 and 26 years of age should consider HPV vaccination with Gardasil. The use of latex condoms has been associated with a decreased risk, not an increased risk, of cervical cancer.

4. **Answer: d**
RATIONALE: The nurse should counsel the client taking metronidazole to avoid alcohol during the treatment because mixing the two causes severe nausea and vomiting. Avoiding extremes of temperature to the genital area is a requirement for clients with genital ulcers, not trichomoniasis. The nurse should instruct the client to avoid sex, regardless of using condoms, until she and her sex partners are cured, i.e., when therapy has been completed and both partners are symptom-free. It is not required to increase fluid intake during treatment.

5. **Answer: a**
RATIONALE: Symptoms of bacterial vaginosis include a characteristic "stale fish" odor and thin, white homogeneous vaginal discharge, not heavy yellow discharge. Dysfunctional uterine bleeding is a sign of chlamydia, not bacterial vaginosis. Erythema in the vulvovaginal area is a symptom of vulvovaginal candidiasis, not bacterial vaginosis.

6. **Answer: d**
RATIONALE: Genital herpes simplex is characterized by lesions, frequently located on the vulva, vagina, and perineal areas. Rashes on the face are not symptoms of HSV. Alopecia is one of the symptoms of syphilis, not of primary HSV. Vaginal discharge during the primary stage of herpes is mucopurulent, not yellow-green.

7. **Answer: c**
RATIONALE: As a nursing strategy to prevent the spread of STIs, the nurse should discuss reducing the number of sex partners to diminish the risk of acquiring STIs. Oral contraceptives are not effective in preventing STIs, and barrier methods (condoms, diaphragms) should be promoted. The nurse should counsel and encourage sex partners of persons with STIs to seek treatment. Maintaining good body hygiene or not sharing personal items with others does not reduce the risk of spreading sexually transmitted infections.

8. **Answer: b**
RATIONALE: The nurse should instruct all community members to get vaccinated for prevention of hepatitis B. Ensuring that drinking water is disease-free and educating people about the risks involved with injecting drugs may help prevent hepatitis A, not hepatitis B. Delaying the start of sexual activity by teenagers may not protect them from hepatitis B in the long run.

9. **Answer: a**
RATIONALE: Although the reasons for bacterial vaginosis are not yet fully understood, sex with multi-ple partners increases the risk, and therefore it should be avoided. Using oral contraceptives and smoking have not been associated with bacterial vaginosis. A colposcopy test is recommended for clients with high-risk HPV, not for diagnosing bacterial vaginosis.

10. **Answer: c**
RATIONALE: The nurse should inform the client that there is no evidence to suggest that antiviral therapy is completely safe during pregnancy. HSV cannot be cured completely, even with timely antiviral drug therapy, and there may be recurrences. The viral shedding process continues for 2 weeks during the primary episode, and kissing during this period may transmit the disease. Recurrent HSV infection episodes are shorter and milder.

11. **Answer: b, c, & e**
RATIONALE: The nurse should instruct the client with pelvic inflammatory disease to avoid douching, limit the number of sex partners, and complete the antibiotic therapy. Use of an intrauterine device is one of the risk factors associated with PID and should be avoided. Increasing fluid intake does not help alleviate the client's condition.

12. **Answer: a, c, & d**
RATIONALE: The nurse should instruct the client to wear nonconstricting clothes and to wash her hands with soap and water after touching lesions to avoid autoinoculation. If urination is painful because of the ulcers, instruct the client to urinate in water but to avoid extremes of temperature such as ice packs or hot pads to the genital area. The client should abstain from intercourse during the prodromal period and when lesions are present. The ulcer disappears during the latency period.

13. **Answer: a, b, & c**
RATIONALE: The nurse should give opportunities to practice negotiation techniques and encourage women to develop refusal skills so that they can respond positively in situations where they might be at risk for HIV infection. To reduce risk of HIV infection, the nurse should encourage the use of female condoms. Supporting youth development activities to reduce sexual risk-taking and identifying or encouraging women to lead a healthy lifestyle may not be effective enough in empowering women to develop control over their lives.

14. **Answer: c, d, & e**
RATIONALE: The nurse should ensure that the client understands the dosing regimen and schedule. The client should be informed that unpleasant side effects such as nausea and diarrhea are common. The nurse should provide written material describing diet, exercise, and medications to promote compliance and ensure a healthy lifestyle. There is no evidence to suggest that exposure of the fetus to antiretroviral agents during pregnancy is completely safe in the long run. HIV is a life-long condition and antiretroviral therapy may delay the onset of AIDS but not prevent it.

15 Answer: b, d, & e

RATIONALE: When educating the client about cervical cancer, the nurse should inform the client that recurrence of genital warts increases the risk of cervical cancer and she should obtain regular Pap smears to detect cervical cancer. Use of latex condoms reduces the risk of cervical cancer. Abnormal vaginal discharge does not necessarily indicate cervical cancer. There is no significant link between use of broad-spectrum antibiotics and increased risk of cervical cancer.

16. Answer: b

RATIONALE: The hepatitis B vaccine consists of a series of three injections given within 6 months. The vaccine is safe and well-tolerated by most babies, including those who are underweight or premature. Vaccines are given after birth in most hospitals, not 6 months later. All babies are vaccinated, not just those whose mothers are identified as at high risk for hepatitis.

17. Answer: b

RATIONALE: To prevent gonococcal ophthalmia neonatorum in the baby, the nurse should instill a prophylactic agent in the eyes of the newborn. Cephalosporins are administered to the mother during pregnancy to treat gonorrhea but not to prevent infection in the newborn. Performing a cesarean operation will not prevent gonococcal ophthalmia neonatorum in the newborn. An antiretroviral syrup is administered to the newborn only if the mother is HIV-positive and will not help prevent gonococcal ophthalmia neonatorum in the baby.

18. Answer: d

RATIONALE: Antiretroviral syrup is administered to the infant within 12 hours after birth to reduce the risk of transmission of HIV to the baby. Delivering the baby via cesarean does not significantly lower the risk of transmitting AIDS to the baby. A triple-combination HAART is used to treat HIV in adults, not babies. The nurse should counsel the client to avoid breastfeeding and use formula instead, because HIV can be spread to the infant through breastfeeding.

CHAPTER 6

Activity A

1. Ultrasound
2. Brachytherapy
3. estrogen
4. Lumpectomy
5. Mammography
6. Chemotherapy
7. mastectomy
8. Hemoccult
9. Immunotherapy
10. Fibroadenomas

Activity B

1. **a.** The disease is known as mastitis, which is an infection of the connective tissue in the breast that occurs primarily in lactating or engorged women.
   b. The clinical manifestations of mastitis are flulike symptoms of malaise, leukocytosis, fever, and chills. Physical examination of the breasts reveals increased warmth, redness, tenderness, and swelling. The nipple is usually cracked or abraded and the breast is distended with milk.
2. **a.** A, fibrocystic breast changes; B, cysts in the later stages
   b. A, fibrocystic breast changes are characterized by fibrosis, or thickening of the normal breast tissues, which occurs in the early stages; B, cysts form in the later stages and feel like multiple, smooth, well-delineated tiny pebbles or bumpy oatmeal under the skin. These cysts tend to be mobile and tender and do not cause skin retraction in the surrounding tissue.

Activity C

1. e   **2.** d   **3.** c   **4.** b   **5.** a

Activity D

1. A benign breast disorder is any noncancerous breast abnormality. Though not life-threatening, benign disorders can cause pain and discomfort and account for a large number of visits to primary care providers. The most commonly encountered benign breast disorders in women include fibrocystic breasts, fibroadenomas, intraductal papilloma, mammary duct ectasia, and mastitis.
2. The three aspects on which breast cancers are classified are tumor size, extent of lymph node involvement, and evidence of metastasis.
3. Breast-conserving surgery, the least invasive procedure, is the wide local excision (or lumpectomy) of the tumor along with a 1-cm margin of normal tissue. A lumpectomy is often used for early-stage localized tumors. The goal of breast-conserving surgery is to remove the suspicious mass along with tissue free of malignant cells to prevent recurrence. The results are less drastic and emotionally less scarring to the woman. Women undergoing breast-conserving therapy receive radiation after lumpectomy with the goal of eradicating residual microscopic cancer cells to limit locoregional recurrence. In women who do not require adjuvant chemotherapy, radiation therapy typically begins 2 to 4 weeks after surgery to allow healing of the lumpectomy incision site. Radiation is administered to the entire breast at daily doses over a period of several weeks.
4. Adjunct therapy is supportive or additional therapy that is recommended after surgery. Adjunct therapies include local therapy such as radiation therapy and systemic therapies such as chemotherapy, hormonal therapy, and immunotherapy.

5. The typical side effects of chemotherapy include nausea and vomiting, diarrhea, or constipation.
6. The status of the axillary lymph nodes is an important prognostic indicator in early-stage breast cancer. The presence or absence of malignant cells in lymph nodes is highly significant. The more lymph nodes involved and the more aggressive the cancer, the more powerful chemotherapy will have to be, in terms of both the toxicity of drugs and the duration of treatment.

Activity E

1. **a.** The nurse should ask the following questions:
   - Where is the lump located, and is it freely moveable or fixed?
   - Does the client have any nipple discharge? If yes, describe its color and consistency.
   - Does the client have a feeling of fullness in the breast?
   - Is the pain dull, burning, or itchy?
   - Is there any skin dimpling or nipple retraction?
   b. Mrs. Taylor needs the following education regarding breast health:
   - Monthly breast self-examination
   - Yearly clinical breast examination
   - Yearly mammography
   c. The treatment modalities available to Mrs. Taylor in case of a malignancy are:
   - Local treatments such as surgery, and radiation
   - Systemic treatments such as chemotherapy, hormonal therapy, and immunotherapy
   d. Mrs. Taylor will need the following community referrals:
   - Telephone counseling by the nurse
   - ACS's Reach for Recovery
   - Organizations or charities that support cancer research
   - Participation in breast cancer walks to raise awareness
   - Emotional support groups

Activity F

1. **Answer: c**
   RATIONALE: During menstrual cycles, hormonal stimulation of the breast tissue causes the glands and ducts to enlarge and swell. The breasts feel swollen, tender, and lumpy during this time, but after menses the swelling and lumpiness decline. This is why it is best to examine the breasts a week after the menses, when they are not swollen. For determining fibrocystic breast changes, it is not best to schedule the breast examination in the second phase of menstrual cycle or immediately after the client has completed her menses.

2. **Answer: b**
   RATIONALE: Since the physician suspects fibroadenomas, it is important for the nurse to know if the client is pregnant or lactating since the incidence of fibroadenomas is more frequent among pregnant and lactating women. Taking oral contraceptives assists a client with fibrocystic breast changes but is not necessary for a client with fibroadenomas. Fibroadenomas usually occur in women between 20 and 30 years of age. Smoking and a high-fat diet will make the client more susceptible to cancer, not fibroadenomas.

3. **Answer: a**
   RATIONALE: The nurse should instruct the client with mastitis to increase her fluid intake. A client with mastitis is instructed to continue breastfeeding as tolerated and to frequently change positions while nursing. The nurse should also instruct the client to apply warm, not cold, compresses to the affected breast area or to take a warm shower before breastfeeding.

4. **Answer: b**
   RATIONALE: When preparing a client for mammography, the nurse should ensure the client has not applied deodorant or powder on the day of testing because they can appear on the x-ray film as calcium spots. It is not necessary for the client to avoid fluid intake an hour prior to testing. Mammography has to be scheduled just after the client's menses to reduce chances of breast tenderness, not when the client is going to start her menses. The client can take aspirin or Tylenol after the completion of the procedure to ease any discomfort, but these medications are not taken before mammography.

5. **Answer: d**
   RATIONALE: The side effects of chemotherapy are constipation, hair loss, weight loss, vomiting, diarrhea, immunosuppression, and, in extreme cases, bone marrow suppression. The nurse should monitor for these side effects when caring for the client undergoing chemotherapy. Vaginal discharge, headache, and chills are not side effects of chemotherapy. Vaginal discharge is one of the side effects of SERMs (selective estrogen receptor modulators) as a part of hormonal therapy, which is used to prevent cancer from spreading further into the body. Headache is a side effect of aromatase inhibitors under hormonal therapy to counter cancer. Chills are a side effect of immunotherapy.

6. **Answer: d**
   RATIONALE: The nurse should inform the client that intraductal papillomas and fibrocystic breasts, although considered benign, carry a cancer risk with prolific masses and hyperplastic changes within the breasts. Other benign breast disorders such as mastitis, mammary duct ectasia, and fibroadenomas carry little risk.

7. **Answer: a**
   RATIONALE: The nurse should inform the client that removing only the sentinel lymph node prevents side effects such as lymphedema, which is otherwise associated with a traditional axillary lymph node dissection. It does not help reveal the hormonal status of the cancer. Hormone-receptor status can be revealed through normal breast

epithelium, which has hormone receptors and responds specifically to the stimulatory effects of estrogen and progesterone. A sentinel lymph node biopsy will determine how powerful a chemotherapy regimen the client will have to undergo, but undergoing a sentinel lymph node biopsy will not lessen the aggressiveness of the chemotherapy. Degree of HER-2/neu oncoprotein will be revealed through the HER-2/neu genetic marker, not through a sentinel lymph node biopsy.

8. **Answer: b**
RATIONALE: When providing care to the client, the nurse should instruct the client to elevate the affected arm on a pillow. As part of the respiratory care, the nurse should instruct the client to turn, cough, and breathe deeply every 2 hours; rapid breathing is not encouraged. Active range-of-motion and arm exercises are necessary. To counter any pain experienced by the client, analgesics are administered as needed; intake of medication is not restricted.

9. **Answer: c**
RATIONALE: Skin edema, redness, and warmth of the breast are symptoms of inflammatory breast cancer. Induced discharge is an indication of benign breast conditions, which are noncancerous. Cancer involves spontaneous nipple discharge. Papillomas and palpable mobile cysts are characteristics of fibroadenomas, intraductal papilloma, and mammary duct ectasia, which are benign breast conditions and are noncancerous.

10. **Answer: d**
RATIONALE: The symptom of mammary duct ectasia that the nurse should assess for is the presence of green, brown, straw-colored, reddish, gray, or cream-colored nipple discharge with a consistency of toothpaste. Increased warmth of the breasts along with redness is a manifestation of mastitis but not mammary duct ectasia. Skin retractions on pulling are a sign of cancer, not mammary duct ectasia. The nurse has to observe nipple retraction. Tortuous tubular swellings are found only beneath the areola, not in the upper half of the breast, in mammary duct ectasia.

11. **Answer: c**
RATIONALE: When caring for a client who is being administered selective estrogen receptor modulator, the nurse should monitor for side effects such as hot flashes, vaginal discharge, bleeding, and cataract formation. Weight loss is one of the side effects of chemotherapy, and fever and chills are the side effects of immunotherapy, not of SERM.

12. **Answer: a, c, & d**
RATIONALE: The modifiable risk factors for breast cancer are postmenopausal use of estrogen and progestins, not having children until after the age of 30, and failing to breastfeed for up to a year after pregnancy. Early menarche or late menopause and previous abnormal breast biopsy are the nonmodifiable risk factors for breast cancer.

13. **Answer: d**
RATIONALE: When performing the breast self-examination, the nurse should instruct the client to apply hard pressure down to the ribs. Light, not medium, pressure should be applied when moving the skin without moving the tissue underneath. Medium, not light, pressure should be applied midway into the tissue. Client need not specifically palpate the areolar area during breast self-examination.

14. **Answer: b**
RATIONALE: Adverse effects of trastuzumab include cardiac toxicity, vascular thrombosis, hepatic failure, fever, chills, nausea, vomiting, and pain with first infusion. The nurse should monitor for these adverse effects with the first infusion of trastuzumab. Dyspnea, stroke, and myelosuppression are not side effects caused with the first infusion of trastuzumab. Dyspnea is a side effect of aromatase inhibitors as part of hormonal therapy. Stroke is an adverse effect of selective estrogen receptive modulator (SERM), again as part of hormonal therapy. Myelosuppression is an extreme side effect of chemotherapy.

15 **Answer: a**
RATIONALE: A nurse should closely monitor for signs of anorexia since it is a likely side effect of radiation therapy, along with swelling and heaviness of the breast, local edema, inflammation, and sunburn-like skin changes. Infection, fever, and nausea are not the side effects of radiation therapy. Infection and fever are the side effects of brachytherapy. Nausea is one of the side effects of chemotherapy.

16. **Answer: b**
RATIONALE: When caring for a client who has just undergone surgery for intraductal papilloma, the nurse should instruct the client to continue monthly breast self-examinations along with yearly clinical breast examinations. Applying warm compresses to the affected breast and wearing a supportive bra 24 hours a day are instructions given in cases of mastitis but not for intraductal papilloma. The nurse should instruct clients to refrain from consuming salt in the diet in cases of fibrocystic breast changes but not in cases of intraductal papilloma.

17. **Answer: b, d, & e**
RATIONALE: Lumpectomy is contraindicated for women who have previously undergone radiation to their affected breast, those whose connective tissue is reported to be sensitive to radiation, and those whose surgery will not result in a clean margin of tissue. Clients who have had an early menarche or late onset of menopause and clients who have failed to breastfeed for up to a year after pregnancy are at risk for developing breast cancer. Lumpectomy is a treatment option for clients with breast cancer.

18. Answer: a, b, & d

RATIONALE: The client is more susceptible to lymphedema if the affected arm is used for drawing blood or measuring blood pressure, if she engages in activities like gardening without using gloves, or if she's not wearing a well-fitted compression sleeve to promote drainage return. Consuming foods rich in phytochemicals is essential to prevent the incidence of cancer, not lymphedema. Not consuming a diet high in fiber and protein will not make the client susceptible to lymphedema.

19. Answer: b, d, & e

RATIONALE: The nurse should instruct the client with fibrocystic breast changes to avoid caffeine. Caffeine acts as a stimulant that can lead to discomfort. It is important to maintain a low-fat diet rich in fruits, vegetables, and grains to maintain a healthy body weight. Taking diuretics is important to counteract fluid retention and swelling of the breasts. Practicing good hand-washing techniques and increasing fluid intake are important for clients with mastitis but may not help clients with fibrocystic breast changes.

20. Answer: a, b, & c

RATIONALE: The nurse should instruct the client to restrict intake of salted foods, limit intake of processed foods, and consume seven or more daily portions of complex carbohydrates, not proteins. Increasing liquid intake to 3 liters daily will not reduce her risk of developing breast cancer.

CHAPTER 7

Activity A

1. Cystocele
2. prolapse
3. pessary
4. Polyps
5. leiomyomas
6. Kegel
7. rectum
8. urethra
9. Metrorrhagia
10. Transvaginal

Activity B

1. The figure shows uterine prolapse, which occurs when the uterus descends through the pelvic floor and into the vaginal canal.
2. The figure shows submucosal, intramural, and subserosal fibroids.

Activity C

1. a **2.** e **3.** b **4.** c **5.** d

Activity D

1. Pelvic organ prolapse could be caused by the following:
   - Constant downward gravity because of erect human posture

   - Atrophy of supporting tissues with aging and decline of estrogen levels
   - Weakening of pelvic support related to childbirth trauma
   - Reproductive surgery
   - Family history of pelvic organ prolapse
   - Young age at first birth
   - Connective tissue disorders
   - Infant birth weight of greater than 4500 grams
   - Pelvic radiation
   - Increased abdominal pressure secondary to lifting of children or heavy objects, straining due to chronic constipation, respiratory problems or chronic coughing, or obesity

2. Kegel exercises strengthen the pelvic-floor muscles to support the inner organs and prevent further prolapse. They help increase the muscle volume, which will result in a stronger muscular contraction. These exercises might limit the progression of mild prolapse and alleviate mild prolapse symptoms, including low back pain and pelvic pressure. Clients with severe uterine prolapse may not benefit from Kegel exercises.

3. Several factors contribute to urinary incontinence:
   - Intake of fluids, especially alcohol, carbonated drinks, and caffeinated beverages
   - Constipation, which alters the position of pelvic organs and puts pressure on the bladder
   - Habitual preventive emptying, which may result in training the bladder to hold small amounts of urine
   - Anatomic changes due to advanced age, which decrease pelvic support
   - Pregnancy and childbirth, which cause damage to the pelvis structure during birthing process
   - Obesity, which increases abdominal pressure

4. The Colpexin Sphere is a polycarbonate sphere with a locator string that is fitted above the hymenal ring to support the pelvis floor muscle. The sphere is used in conjunction with pelvic floor muscle exercises, which should be performed daily. The sphere supports the pelvic floor muscle and facilitates rehabilitation of the pelvic floor muscles.

5. Uterine fibroids may be medically managed by uterine artery embolization (UAE). UAE is an option in which polyvinyl alcohol pellets are injected into selected blood vessels via a catheter to block circulation to the fibroid, causing shrinkage of the fibroid and resolution of the symptoms. After treatment, most fibroids are reduced by 50% within 3 months, but they might recur. The failure rate is approximately 10% to 15%, and this therapy should not be performed on women desiring to retain their fertility.

6. Bartholin's glands are two mucus-secreting glandular structures with duct openings bilaterally at the base of the labia minora, near the opening of the vagina, that provide lubrication during sexual arousal. A Bartholin's cyst is a fluid-filled, swollen, saclike structure that results from a blockage of one

of the ducts of the Bartholin gland. The cyst may become infected and an abscess may develop in the gland. Bartholin's cysts are the most common cystic growths in the vulva, affecting approximately 2% of women at some time in their lives.

Activity E

1. **a.** Pelvic support disorders increase with age and are a result of weakness of the connective tissue and muscular support of the pelvic organs. Vaginal childbirth, obesity, lifting, chronic cough, straining at defecation secondary to constipation, and estrogen deficiency all contribute to pelvic support disorders.
   b. Symptoms of uterine prolapse include low back pain, pelvic pressure, urinary frequency, retention, and/or incontinence. These symptoms are likely to affect Mrs. Scott's daily activities.
   c. Nonsurgical interventions include regular Kegel exercises, estrogen replacement therapy, dietary and lifestyle modifications, and pessaries. Kegel exercises might limit the progression of mild prolapse and alleviate mild prolapse symptoms, including low back pain and pelvic pressure. Estrogen replacement therapy may help to improve the tone and vascularity of the supporting tissue in perimenopausal and menopausal women by increasing blood perfusion and elasticity to the vaginal wall. Dietary and lifestyle modifications may help prevent pelvic relaxation and chronic problems later in life. Pessaries may be indicated for uterine prolapse or cystocele, especially among elderly clients for whom surgery is contraindicated. Surgical interventions include anterior and posterior colporrhaphy and vaginal hysterectomy. Anterior and posterior colporrhaphy may be effective for a first-degree prolapse. A vaginal hysterectomy is the treatment of choice for uterine prolapse because it removes the prolapsed organ that is bringing down the bladder and rectum with it.

Activity F

1. **Answer: c**
   RATIONALE: Weakening of the pelvic-floor muscles causes a feeling of dragging and a "lump" in the vagina; these are symptoms of pelvic organ prolapse. These symptoms do not indicate urinary incontinence, endocervical polyps, or uterine fibroids. Urinary incontinence is the involuntary loss of urine. The symptoms of endocervical polyps are abnormal vaginal bleeding or discharge. In cases of uterine fibroids, the uterus is enlarged and irregularly shaped.

2. **Answer: b**
   RATIONALE: Before starting estrogen replacement therapy, each woman must be evaluated on the basis of a thorough medical history to validate her risk for complications such as endometrial cancer, myocardial infarction, stroke, breast cancer, pul-

monary emboli, or deep vein thrombosis. The effective dose of estrogen required, the dietary modifications, and the cost of estrogen replacement therapy can be discussed at a later stage when the client understands the risks associated with estrogen replacement therapy and decides to use hormone therapy.

3. **Answer: a**
   RATIONALE: The nurse should instruct the client to increase dietary fiber and fluids to prevent constipation. A high-fiber diet with an increase in fluid intake alleviates constipation by increasing stool bulk and stimulating peristalsis. Straining to pass a hard stool increases intra-abdominal pressure, which, over time, causes the pelvic organs to prolapse. Avoiding caffeine products would not help substantially; instead, the client should give up smoking to minimize the risk for a chronic "smoker's cough." In addition to recommending increasing the amount of fiber in her diet, the nurse should also encourage the woman to drink eight 8-oz glasses of fluid daily. The nurse should instruct the client to avoid high-impact aerobics to minimize the risk of increasing intra-abdominal pressure.

4. **Answer: d**
   RATIONALE: The disadvantage of myomectomy is that the fibroids may grow back in the future. Fertility is not jeopardized, because this procedure leaves the uterine wall intact. Weakening of the uterine walls, scarring, and adhesions are caused by laser treatment, not myomectomy.

5. **Answer: b**
   RATIONALE: Kegel exercises might limit the progression of mild prolapse and alleviate mild prolapse symptoms, including low back pain and pelvic pressure. Intake of food is not required before performing Kegel exercises. Surgical interventions do not interfere with Kegel exercises. Kegel exercises do not cause an increase in blood pressure.

6. **Answer: a, b, & d**
   RATIONALE: The predisposing factors for uterine fibroids are age (late reproductive years), nulliparity, obesity, genetic predisposition, and African-American ethnicity. Smoking and hyperinsulinemia are not predisposing factors for uterine fibroids.

7. **Answer: b**
   RATIONALE: Vaginal dryness is one of the side effects of GnRH medications. The other side effects of GnRH medications are hot flashes, headaches, mood changes, musculoskeletal malaise, bone loss, and depression. Increased vaginal discharge, urinary tract infections, and vaginitis are side effects of a pessary, not GnRH medications.

8. **Answer: c**
   RATIONALE: The nurse should instruct the client using a pessary to report any discomfort or difficulty with urination or defecation. Avoiding high-impact aerobics, jogging, jumping, and

lifting heavy objects, as well as wearing a girdle or abdominal support, are recommended for a client with prolapse as part of lifestyle modifications and may not be necessary for a client using a pessary.

9. **Answer: b**
RATIONALE: The most common recommendation for pessary care is removing the pessary twice weekly and cleaning it with soap and water. In addition, douching with diluted vinegar or hydrogen peroxide helps to reduce urinary tract infections and odor, which are side effects of using a pessary. Estrogen cream is applied to make the vaginal mucosa more resistant to erosion and strengthen the vaginal walls. Removing the pessary before sleeping or intercourse is not part of the instructions for pessary care.

10. **Answer: d**
RATIONALE: The nurse should monitor the client with ultrasound scans every 3 to 6 months. Monitoring gonadotropin level and blood sugar level and scheduling periodic Pap smears are not important assessments for the client with small ovarian cysts.

11. **Answer: a**
RATIONALE: The nurse should teach the client turning, deep breathing, and coughing prior to the surgery to prevent atelectasis and respiratory complications such as pneumonia. Reducing activity level and the need for pelvic rest are instructions related to discharge planning after the client has undergone a hysterectomy. A high-fat diet need not be avoided before undergoing hysterectomy; avoiding a high-fat diet is required for clients with pelvic organ prolapse to reduce constipation.

12. **Answer: b, c, & e**
RATIONALE: If the client is at high risk of recurrent prolapse after a surgical repair, is morbidly obese, or has chronic obstructive pulmonary disease, then the client is not a good candidate for surgical repair. Low back pain and pelvic pressure are common to almost all pelvic organ prolapses and do not help to decide whether the client should opt for surgical repair. A client with severe pelvic organ prolapse may be a candidate for surgical repair.

13. **Answer: a, b, & d**
RATIONALE: The teaching guidelines include continuing pelvic floor (Kegel) exercises, increasing fiber in the diet to reduce constipation, and controlling blood glucose levels to prevent polyuria. The nurse should instruct the client to reduce the intake of fluids and foods that are bladder irritants, such as orange juice, soda, and caffeine, and the client should wipe from front to back to prevent urinary tract infections.

14. **Answer: a, d, & e**
RATIONALE: The postoperative care plan for a client who has undergone a hysterectomy includes administering analgesics promptly and using a PCA pump, changing linens and gown frequently to promote hygiene, and administering antiemetics to control nausea and vomiting. The nurse should change the position of the client frequently and use pillows for support to promote comfort and pain management. An excess of carbonated beverages in the diet does not affect the postoperative healing process.

15. **Answer: a**
RATIONALE: The nurse should stress follow-up care to the client with polycystic ovarian syndrome so that the client does not overlook this benign disorder. Increasing intake of fiber-rich foods, increasing fluid intake, and performing Kegel exercises help to control pelvic organ prolapse, not PCOS.

CHAPTER 8

Activity A

1. dysplasia
2. Colposcopy
3. Cryotherapy
4. Endometrial
5. Bethesda
6. Hysterectomy
7. CA-125
8. simplex
9. epithelium
10. Squamous

Activity B

1. a. The image shows ovarian cancer.
   b. The treatment options available for ovarian cancer are as follows:
   - Surgery includes a total abdominal hysterectomy, bilateral salpingo-oophorectomy, peritoneal biopsies, omentectomy, and pelvic para-aortic lymph node sampling to evaluate cancer extension.
   - Aggressive management involving debulking or cytoreductive surgery is commonly performed for advanced-stage ovarian cancer.
   - Additional therapy with radiation may be warranted.
   - Chemotherapy is recommended for all stages of ovarian cancer.
2. a. The image shows vulvar cancer.
   b. Treatment for vulvar cancer varies, depending on the extent of the disease. Laser surgery, cryosurgery, or electrosurgical incision may be used. Larger lesions may need more extensive surgery and skin grafting. The traditional treatment for vulvar cancer has been radical vulvectomy, but more conservative techniques are being used to improve psychosexual outcomes.

Activity C

1. b   2. a   3. d   4. c

Activity D

1.

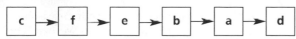

c → f → e → b → a → d

Activity E

1. Risk factors for developing cervical cancer are as follows:
   - Early age of first intercourse (within 1 year of menarche)
   - Lower socioeconomic status
   - Promiscuous male partners
   - Unprotected sexual intercourse
   - Family history of cervical cancer (mother or sisters)
   - Sexual intercourse with uncircumcised men
   - Female offspring of mothers who took diethylstilbestrol (DES)
   - Infections with genital herpes or chronic chlamydia
   - History of multiple sex partners
   - Cigarette smoking
   - Immunocompromised state
   - HIV infection
   - Oral contraceptive use
   - Moderate dysplasia on Pap smear within past 5 years
   - HPV infection
2. Treatment options for endometrial cancer are as follows:
   - Treatment of endometrial cancer depends on the stage of the disease and usually involves surgery, with adjunct therapy based on pathologic findings.
   - Surgery most often involves removal of the uterus (hysterectomy) and the fallopian tubes and ovaries (salpingo-oophorectomy).
   - In more advanced cancers, radiation and chemotherapy are used as adjunct therapies to surgery.
   - Routine surveillance intervals for follow-up care are typically every 3 to 4 months for the first 2 years, since 85% of recurrences occur in the first two years after diagnosis.
3. The following are possible risk factors for ovarian cancer:
   - Nulliparity
   - Early menarche (<12 years old)
   - Late menopause (>55 years old)
   - Increasing age (>50 years of age)
   - High-fat diet
   - Obesity
   - Persistent ovulation over time
   - First-degree relative with ovarian cancer
   - Use of perineal talcum powder or hygiene sprays
   - Older than 30 years at first pregnancy
   - Positive BRCA-1 and BRCA-2 mutations
   - Personal history of breast, bladder, or colon cancer
   - Hormone replacement therapy for more than 10 years
   - Infertility
4. Transvaginal ultrasound can be used to evaluate the endometrial cavity and measure the thickness of the endometrial lining. It can be used to detect endometrial hyperplasia.
5. The following are the nursing interventions in caring for clients with cancers of the female reproductive tract:
   - Validate the client's feelings and provide realistic hope.
   - Use basic communication skills in a sincere way during all interactions.
   - Provide useful, nonjudgmental information to all women.
   - Individualize care to address the client's cultural traditions.
   - Carry out postoperative care and instructions as prescribed.
   - Discuss postoperative issues, including incision care, pain, and activity level.
   - Instruct the client on health maintenance activities after treatment.
   - Inform the client and family about available support resources.
6. The following are the diagnostic options for endometrial cancer:
   - Endometrial biopsy: An endometrial biopsy is the procedure of choice to make the diagnosis. It can be done in the health care provider's office without anesthesia. A slender suction catheter is used to obtain a small sample of tissue for pathology. It can detect up to 90% of cases of endometrial cancer in the woman with postmenopausal bleeding, depending on the technique and experience of the health care provider. The woman may experience mild cramping and bleeding after the procedure for about 24 hours, but typically mild pain medication will reduce this discomfort.
   - Transvaginal ultrasound: A transvaginal ultrasound can be used to evaluate the endometrial cavity and measure the thickness of the endometrial lining. It can be used to detect endometrial hyperplasia. If the endometrium measures less than 4 mm, then the client is at low risk for malignancy.

Activity F

1. a.
   - Back pain
   - Abdominal bloating
   - Fatigue
   - Urinary frequency
   - Constipation
   - Abdominal pressure
   b. The most common early symptoms include abdominal bloating, early satiety, fatigue, vague abdominal pain, urinary frequency, diarrhea or constipation, and unexplained weight loss or

gain. The later symptoms include anorexia, dyspepsia, ascites, palpable abdominal mass, pelvic pain, and back pain. Early detection of ovarian cancer is possible if the clients are informed about yearly bimanual pelvic examination and transvaginal ultrasound to identify ovarian masses.

c. Disturbed body image related to:
  • Loss of body part
  • Loss of good health
  • Altered sexuality patterns
  Anxiety related to:
  • Threat of malignancy
  • Potential diagnosis
  • Anticipated pain/discomfort
  • Effect of condition treatment on future
  Deficient knowledge related to:
  • Disease process and prognosis
  • Specific treatment options
  • Diagnostic procedures needed

d. In Stage I, the ovarian cancer is limited to the ovaries. In Stage II, the growth involves one or both ovaries, with pelvic extension. In Stage III, the cancer spreads to the lymph nodes and other organs or structures inside the abdominal cavity. In Stage IV, the cancer has metastasized to distant sites. Treatment options for ovarian cancer vary, depending on the stage and severity of the disease. Usually a laparoscopy (abdominal exploration with an endoscope) is performed for diagnosis and staging, as well as evaluation for further therapy.

Activity G

1. **Answer: a**
RATIONALE: The client should have Papanicolaou tests regularly to detect cervical cancer during the early stages. Blood tests for mutations in the BRCA genes indicate the lifetime risk of the client of developing breast or ovarian cancer. CA-125 is a biologic tumor marker associated with ovarian cancer, but it is not currently sensitive enough to serve as a screening tool.

2. **Answer: a**
RATIONALE: Early onset of sexual activity, within the first year of menarche, increases the risk of acquiring cervical cancer later on. Obesity, infertility, and hypertension are risk factors that are associated with endometrial cancer.

3. **Answer: c**
RATIONALE: The nurse should inform the client that surgery most often involves removal of the uterus (hysterectomy) and the fallopian tubes and ovaries (salpingo-oophorectomy). Removal of the tubes and ovaries, not just the uterus, is recommended because tumor cells spread early to the ovaries, and any dormant cancer cells could be stimulated to grow by ovarian estrogen. In advanced cancers, radiation and chemotherapy are used as adjuvant therapies to surgery. Routine surveillance intervals

for follow-up care are typically every 3 to 4 months for the first 2 years.

4. **Answer: b**
RATIONALE: The client's present age increases her risk of developing ovarian cancer, as women who are older than 50 are at a greater risk. The client's age at menarche (older than 12) and menopause (younger than 55) are both normal. The client is underweight and not obese, so her weight is not a risk factor for ovarian cancer.

5. **Answer: c**
RATIONALE: To identify ovarian masses in their early stages, the client needs to have yearly bimanual pelvic examinations and a transvaginal ultrasound. Pap smears are not effective enough to detect ovarian masses. The U.S. Preventive Services Task Force (USPSTF) recommends against routine screening for ovarian cancer with serum CA-125, because the potential harm could outweigh the potential benefits. X-rays of the pelvic area do not detect ovarian masses.

6. **Answer: a**
RATIONALE: Only 5% of ovarian cancers are genetic in origin. However, the nurse needs to tell the client to seek genetic counseling and thorough assessment to reduce her risk of ovarian cancer. Oral contraceptives reduce the risk of ovarian cancer and should be encouraged. Breastfeeding should be encouraged as a risk-reducing strategy. The nurse should instruct the client to avoid using perineal talc or hygiene sprays.

7. **Answer: c**
RATIONALE: The nurse should instruct the client to avoid wearing tight, restrictive undergarments. The nurse should teach the client genital self-examination to assess for any unusual growths in the vulvar area. The nurse should instruct the client to seek care for any suspicious lesions and to avoid self-medication. The client should use barrier methods of birth control (such as condoms) to reduce the risk of contracting sexually transmitted infections that may increase the risk of vulvar cancer.

8. **Answer: b, c, & e**
RATIONALE: To reduce the risk of cervical cancer, the nurse should encourage clients to avoid smoking and drinking. In addition, because STIs such as HPV increase the risk of cervical cancers, care should be taken to prevent STIs. Teenagers also should be counseled to avoid early sexual activity, because it increases the risk of cervical cancer. The use of barrier methods of contraception, not IUDs, should be encouraged. Avoiding stress and high blood pressure will not have a significant impact on the risk of cervical cancer.

9. **Answer: a, c, & d**
RATIONALE: The responsibilities of a nurse while caring for a client with endometrial cancer include ensuring that the client understands all the treatment options available, suggesting the advantages of a support group and providing referrals, and

offering the family explanations and emotional support throughout the treatment. The nurse should also discuss changes in sexuality with the client as well as stress the importance of regular follow-up care after the treatment and not just in cases where something unusual occurs.

10. **Answer: b, d, & e**
    RATIONALE: Irregular vaginal bleeding, persistent low backache not related to standing, and elevated or discolored vulvar lesions are some of the symptoms that should be immediately brought to the notice of the primary health care provider. Increase in urinary frequency and irregular bowel movements are not symptoms related to cancers of the reproductive tract.

11. **Answer: b**
    RATIONALE: The nurse should explain to the client that the colposcopy is done because the physician has observed abnormalities in Pap smears. The nurse should also explain to the client that the procedure is painless and there are no adverse effects, such as pain during urination. There is no need to avoid intercourse for a week after the colposcopy.

12. **Answer: b**
    RATIONALE: According to the 2001 Bethesda system for classifying Pap smear results, a result of ASC-H means that the client is to be referred for colposcopy without HPV testing. ASC-US means that the test has to be repeated in 4 to 6 months or the client has to be referred for colposcopy. AGC or AIS results indicate immediate colposcopy, with the follow-up based on the results of findings.

13. **Answer: a**
    RATIONALE: Abnormal and painless vaginal bleeding is a major initial symptom of endometrial cancer. Diabetes mellitus and liver disease are the risk factors, not symptoms, for endometrial cancer. Back pain is associated with ovarian cancer.

14. **Answer: a, b, & d**
    RATIONALE: Although direct risk factors for the initial development of vaginal cancer have not been identified, associated risk factors include advancing age (>60 years old), HIV infection, smoking, previous pelvic radiation, exposure to diethylstilbestrol (DES) in utero, vaginal trauma, history of genital warts (HPV infection), cervical cancer, chronic vaginal discharge, and low socioeconomic level. Persistent ovulation over time and hormone replacement therapy for more than 10 years are risk factors associated with ovarian cancer.

15. **Answer: a**
    RATIONALE: The skin condition Lichen sclerosus has been linked with risk of vulvar cancer. Previous pelvic radiation and exposure to diethylstilbestrol (DES) in utero are risk factors associated with vaginal rather than vulvar cancer, and tamoxifen use is a risk factor for endometrial cancer.

CHAPTER 9

Activity A
1. battered
2. Incest
3. Statutory
4. Rohypnol
5. circumcision
6. Acquaintance
7. sexual
8. hyperarousal
9. avoidance
10. dermoid

Activity B
1. d 2. b 3. a 4. c

Activity C
1.

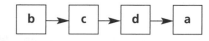

Activity D
1. The cycle of violence occurs in an abusive relationship. It includes three distinct phases: the tension-building phase, the acute battering phase, and the honeymoon phase. The cyclic behavior begins with a time of tension-building arguments, progresses to violence, and settles into a making-up or calm period. With time, this cycle of violence increases in frequency and severity as it is repeated over and over again. The cycle can cover a long or short period of time. The honeymoon phase gradually shortens and eventually disappears altogether.

2. An abuser may financially abuse the partner in the following ways:
   - Preventing the woman from getting a job
   - Sabotaging the current job
   - Controlling how all money is spent
   - Refusing to contribute financially

3. The potential nursing diagnoses related to violence against women include the following:
   - Deficient knowledge related to understanding of the cycle of violence and availability of resources
   - Fear related to possibility of severe injury to self or children during cycle of violence
   - Low self-esteem related to feelings of worthlessness
   - Hopelessness related to prolonged exposure to violence
   - Compromised individual and family coping related to persistence of victim–abuser relationship

4. Posttraumatic stress disorder (PTSD) develops when an event outside the range of normal human experience occurs that produces marked distress in the person. Symptoms of PTSD are divided into 3 groups:
   - Intrusion (re-experiencing the trauma, including nightmares, flashbacks, recurrent thoughts)

- Avoidance (avoiding trauma-related stimuli, social withdrawal, emotional numbing)
- Hyperarousal (increased emotional arousal, exaggerated startle response, irritability)

5. The nurse should screen the client for the following signs to determine if she is a victim of abuse:
   - Injuries: bruises, scars from blunt trauma, or weapon wounds on the face, head, and neck
   - Injury sequelae: headaches, hearing loss, joint pain, sinus infections, teeth marks, clumps of hair missing, dental trauma, pelvic pain, breast or genital injuries
   - The reported history of the injury doesn't seem to add up to the actual presenting problem
   - Mental health problems: depression, anxiety, substance abuse, eating disorders, suicidal ideation, or suicide attempts
   - Frequent health care visits for chronic, stress-related disorders such as chest pain, headaches, back or pelvic pain, insomnia, and gastrointestinal disturbances
   - Partner's behavior at the health care visit: appears overly solicitous or overprotective, unwilling to leave client alone with the health care provider, answers questions for her, and attempts to control the situation in the health care setting

6. Abuse during pregnancy threatens the well-being of the mother and fetus. Physical violence to the pregnant woman brings injuries to the head, face, neck, thorax, breasts, and abdomen. Mental health consequences are also significant. Women assaulted during pregnancy are at a risk for depression, chronic anxiety, insomnia, poor nutrition, excessive weight gain or loss, late entry into prenatal care, preterm labor, miscarriage, stillbirth, premature and low-birth-weight infants, placental abruption, uterine rupture, chorioamnionitis, vaginitis, sexually transmitted infections, urinary tract infections, or smoking and substance abuse.

Activity E

1. **a.** Some of the common symptoms of physical abuse include depression, sexual dysfunction, backaches, sexually transmitted infections, fear or guilt, or phobias.
   b. Suzanne may not seek help in the abusive relationship for the following reasons:
   - She may feel responsible for the abuse.
   - She may feel she deserved the abuse.
   - She may have been abused as a child and has low self-esteem.
   c. The following strategies may help Suzanne to manage the situation:
   - Teaching coping strategies to manage stress
   - Encouraging the establishment of realistic goals
   - Teaching problem-solving skills
   - Encouraging social activities to connect with other people
   - Explaining that abuse is never OK

Activity F

1. **Answer: c**
   RATIONALE: The nurse should inform the client that alcohol, drugs, money problems, depression, or jealousy do not cause violence and are excuses given by the abuser for losing control. Even though violence against women was common in the past, the police, justice system, and society are beginning to make domestic violence socially unacceptable. The nurse also needs to emphasize that physical abuse is not the result of provocation from the female but an expression of inadequacy of the perpetrator. Violence against women is widespread, and whatever the cause of the assault, there is no justification for physical or sexual assault.

2. **Answer: a**
   RATIONALE: The nurse should clearly explain to the client that whatever the cause of the incident, no one deserves to be a victim of physical abuse. Even though the partner appears to be genuinely contrite, most people who attack their spouses are serial abusers and there is no certainty that they will not repeat their actions. The client should realize that even if she tries her best not to upset her partner, her partner may abuse her again. The client should never accept battering as a normal part of any relationship.

3. **Answer: c**
   RATIONALE: Attacking pets and destroying valued possessions are examples of emotional abuse. Observing the client's movements closely may be a sign of suspicion. Throwing objects at the client is physical abuse. Forcing the client to have intercourse against her will is an act of sexual abuse.

4. **Answer: b**
   RATIONALE: Abusers are most likely to exhibit antisocial behavior or childlike aggression. They use aggression to control their victims. Abusers come from all walks of life; they are not just restricted to low-income groups, nor are they necessarily products of divorced parents. The physical characteristics of the abusers vary, and they are not necessarily physically imposing.

5. **Answer: d**
   RATIONALE: For every rape victim who turns up, the nurse should ensure that the appropriate law enforcement agencies are apprised of the incident. Victims should not be made to wait long hours in the waiting room, as they may leave if no one attends to them. Victims of rape should be treated with more sensitivity than other clients. While the primary job of a nurse is to medically care for the rape victim, a nurse should also pay due attention to collecting evidence to substantiate the victim's claim in a court of law.

6. **Answer: c**
   RATIONALE: The nurse should tell the client that she is a victim of sexual abuse because her partner forces her to have intercourse against her will. The

nurse should also explain to the client that she is in no way responsible for such incidents and that she has a right to refuse sexual intimacy. There is no justification for sexual abuse and the client should not regard it as "normal" behavior.

7. **Answer: c**
RATIONALE: The nurse should use pictures and diagrams to ensure that the client understands what is being explained. Instead of using medical terms, the nurse should use simple, accurate terms as much as possible. The nurse should look directly at the client while speaking to her and not at the interpreter. The nurse should not place any judgment on the cultural practice.

8. **Answer: b**
RATIONALE: If the nurse suspects physical abuse, the nurse should attempt to interview the woman in private. Many abusers will not leave their partners for fear of being discovered. The nurse should use subtle ways of doing this, such as telling the woman a urine specimen is required and showing her the way to the restroom, providing the nurse and client some private time. Asking the partner directly if he was responsible will not help because the partner may not admit his culpability. Telling the partner to leave the room immediately may rouse the suspicions of the partner. Questioning the client about the injury in front of the partner may trigger another abusive episode and should be avoided. Precaution should be taken to prevent the abuser from punishing the woman when she returns home.

9. **Answer: a**
RATIONALE: The nurse should use direct quotes and specific language as much as possible when documenting. The nurse should not obtain photos of the client without informed consent. The nurse should, however, document the refusal of the client to be photographed. Documentation must include details as to the frequency and severity of abuse and the location, extent, and outcome of injuries, not just a description of the interventions taken. The nurse is required by law to inform the police of any injuries that involve knives, firearms, or other deadly weapons or that present life-threatening emergencies. Hence, the nurse should explain to the client why the case has to be reported to the police.

10. **Answer: a**
RATIONALE: The nurse should offer referrals to the client, such as support groups or specialists, so that the client gets professional help in recovering from the incident. The nurse should help the client cope with the incident rather than telling the client to forget about it. The nurse should also educate the client about the connection between the violence and some of the symptoms that she has developed recently, like palpitations. Confirming with the partner whether the client's story is true will create further problems for the client, and the nurse may lose the client's trust.

11. **Answer: a**
RATIONALE: To minimize risk of pregnancy, the nurse should ensure that the client takes a double dose of emergency contraceptive pills: the first dose within 72 hours of the rape and the second dose 12 hours after the first dose, if not sooner. It is better to use contraceptive measures immediately than to wait for signs of pregnancy. Using spermicidal creams or gels or regular oral contraceptive pills will not prove effective in preventing unwanted pregnancies.

12. **Answer: b, c, & d**
RATIONALE: Some of the factors that may lead to abuse during pregnancy are resentment toward the interference of the growing fetus and change in the woman's shape, perception of the baby as a competitor once he or she is born, and insecurity and jealousy of the pregnancy and the responsibilities it brings. Concern for the child will never result in physical abuse, as the unborn child is also at risk through assault during pregnancy. Serial abusers may exhibit violent tendencies during pregnancy, and such behavior is unacceptable.

13. **Answer: a, b, & e**
RATIONALE: Victims of human trafficking have restrictions on their daily movements, so the nurse should ask questions to learn whether the client can move around freely. The nurse should also find out if the client could leave her present job or situation if she wants to. Asking clients what their parents do or what their educational background is does not help determine whether they are victims of human trafficking.

14. **Answer: b, c, & e**
RATIONALE: To screen for abuse, the nurse should assess for mental health problems or injuries. The nurse should also be alert for inconsistencies regarding the reporting of the injury and the actual problem. Having sexually transmitted infections frequently is not a sign of physical or sexual abuse. Usually, partners of suspected victims seem overprotective and they do not leave the client alone.

15. **Answer: a, b, & c**
RATIONALE: To learn whether the client is having physical symptoms of PTSD, the nurse should ask the client if she is having trouble sleeping and whether she is emotionally stable or given to bursts of irritability. The nurse should also find out if the client experiences heart palpitations or sweating. Asking the client if she is feeling numb emotionally assesses the presence of avoidance reactions, not physical manifestation of PTSD. The nurse should ask the client whether she has upsetting thoughts and nightmares to assess for the presence of intrusive thoughts.

CHAPTER 10

Activity A

1. Allele
2. mutation
3. autosomes
4. amnion
5. Chromosomes
6. morula
7. karyotype
8. Polyploidy
9. genome
10. phenotype

Activity B

1. The figure shows spermatogenesis. One spermatogonium gives rise to four spermatozoa.
2. The figure shows oogenesis. One mature ovum and three abortive cells are produced from each oogonium.
3. The figure shows fetal circulation. The arrows indicate the path of blood.
4. The umbilical vein carries oxygen-rich blood from the placenta to the liver and through the ductus venosus. From there it is carried to the inferior vena cava to the right atrium of the heart. Some of the blood is shunted through the foramen ovale to the left side of the heart where it is routed to the brain and upper extremities. The rest of the blood travels down to the right ventricle and through the pulmonary artery. A small portion of the blood travels to the non-functioning lungs, while the remaining blood is shunted through the ductus arteriosus into the aorta to supply the rest of the body.

Activity C

1. d   **2.** e   **3.** c   **4.** b   **5.** a

Activity D

1. For conception or fertilization to occur, a healthy ovum from the woman has to be released from the ovary. It passes into an open fallopian tube and starts its journey downward. Sperm from the male must be deposited into the vagina and be able to swim approximately seven inches to meet the ovum where one spermatozoa penetrates the ovum's thick outer membrane. Fertilization takes place in the outer third of the ampulla of the fallopian tube.
2. The three different stages of fetal development during pregnancy are:
   • Preembryonic stage: begins with fertilization through the second week
   • Embryonic stage: begins 15 days after conception and continues through week eight
   • Fetal stage: begins from the end of the eighth week and lasts until birth
3. The sex of the zygote is determined at fertilization. It depends on whether the ovum is fertilized by a Y-bearing sperm or an X-bearing sperm. An XX zygote will become a female, and an XY zygote will become a male.
4. Concurrent with the development of the trophoblast and implantation, further differentiation of the inner cell mass of the zygote occurs. Some of the cells become the embryo itself, and others give rise to the membranes that surround and protect it. The three embryonic layers of cells formed are:
   • Ectoderm—forms the central nervous system, special senses, skin, and glands
   • Mesoderm—forms the skeletal, urinary, circulatory, and reproductive organs
   • Endoderm—forms the respiratory system, liver, pancreas, and digestive system
5. Amniotic fluid is derived from fluid transported from the maternal blood across the amnion and fetal urine. Its volume changes constantly as the fetus swallows and voids. Amniotic fluid is composed of 98% water and 2% organic matter. It is slightly alkaline and contains albumin, urea, uric acid, creatinine, bilirubin, lecithin, sphingomyelin, epithelial cells, vernix, and fine hair called lanugo.
6. The placenta produces hormones that control the basic physiology of the mother in such a way that the fetus is supplied with the necessary nutrients and oxygen needed for successful growth. The placenta produces the following hormones necessary for normal pregnancy:
   • Human chorionic gonadotropin (hCG)
   • Human placental lactogen (hPL)
   • Estrogen (estriol)
   • Progesterone (progestin)
   • Relaxin

Activity E

1. The nurse should explain the following functions of the amniotic fluid:
   • Helps maintain a constant body temperature for the fetus
   • Permits symmetric growth and development of the fetus
   • Cushions the fetus from trauma
   • Allows the umbilical cord to be free of compression
   • Promotes fetal movement to enhance musculoskeletal development
   • Amniotic fluid volume can be important in determining fetal well-being
   The nurse should explain the following functions of the placenta:
   • Makes hormones to ensure implantation of the embryo and to control the mother's physiology to provide adequate nutrients and water to the growing fetus
   • Transports oxygen and nutrients from the mother's bloodstream to the developing fetus
   • Protects the fetus from immune attack by the mother
   • Removes fetal waste products
   • Near term, produces hormones to mature fetal organs in preparation for extrauterine life

The nurse should also explain the following about the umbilical cord:

- The lifeline from the mother to the fetus
- Formed from the amnion and contains one large vein and two small arteries
- Wharton's jelly surrounds the vessels to prevent compression
- At term, the average length is 22 inches long and 1 inch in width

Shana should be reassured that she will continue to feel fetal movement throughout her pregnancy and that it is not common for a fetus to get "tangled in its umbilical cord."

Activity F

1. **Answer: b**
   RATIONALE: This disorder is not X-linked. Either the father or the mother can pass the gene along regardless of whether their mate has the gene or not. The only way that an autosomal dominant gene is not expressed is if it does not exist. If only one of the parents has the gene, then there is a 50% chance it will be passed on to the child.

2. **Answer: c**
   RATIONALE: The nurse should instruct the client to stop using drugs, alcohol, and tobacco, as these harmful substances may be passed on to the fetus from the mother. There is no need to avoid exercise during pregnancy as long as the client follows the prescribed regimen. Wearing comfortable clothes is not as important as the client's health. The client need not stay indoors during pregnancy.

3. **Answer: c**
   RATIONALE: The nurse should find out the age and cause of death for deceased family members, as it will help establish a genetic pattern. Instances of premature birth or depression during pregnancy are not related to any genetically inherited disorders. A family history of drinking or drug abuse does not increase the risk of genetic disorders.

4. **Answer: a**
   RATIONALE: The risk of trisomies such as Klinefelter syndrome increases with the age of the mother at the time of pregnancy. Klinefelter syndrome occurs only in males. Having twins does not increase the risk of Klinefelter syndrome for the babies, nor does the client's previous smoking habit have any bearing on the risk for Klinefelter syndrome.

5. **Answer: b**
   RATIONALE: Down syndrome occurs because of the presence of an extra chromosome in the body. Down syndrome is not genetically inherited. Both males and females are equally at risk for Down syndrome. Most children with Down syndrome have mild to moderate mental retardation.

6. **Answer: d**
   RATIONALE: While obtaining the genetic history of the client, the nurse should find out if the members of the couple are related to each other or have blood ties, as this increases the risk of many genetic disorders. The socioeconomic status or the physical characteristics of family members do not have any significant bearing on the risk of genetic disorders. The nurse should ask questions about race or ethnic background because some races are more susceptible to certain disorders than others.

7. **Answer: c**
   RATIONALE: After the client has seen the specialist, the nurse should review what the specialist has discussed with the family and clarify any doubts the couple may have. The nurse should never make the decision for the client but rather should present all the relevant information and aid the couple in making an informed decision. There is no need for the nurse to refer the client to another specialist or for further diagnostic and screening tests unless instructed to do so by the specialist.

8. **Answer: a**
   RATIONALE: Tay-Sachs disease affects both male and female babies. The age of the client does not significantly increase the risk of Tay-Sachs disease. Even though the client and her husband are not related by blood, because of their background (Ashkenazi heritage) their baby is at a greater risk. There is a chance that the offspring may have Tay-Sachs disease even if both parents don't have it because they could be carriers.

9. **Answer: b, d & e**
   RATIONALE: The nurse should explain to the client that individuals with hemophilia are usually males. Female carriers have a 50% chance of transmitting the disorder to their sons, and females are affected by the condition if it is a dominant X-linked disorder. Offspring of non-hemophilic parents may be hemophilic. Daughters of an affected male are usually carriers.

10. **Answer: a, b, & d**
    RATIONALE: The responsibilities of the nurse while counseling the client include knowing basic genetic terminology and inheritance patterns and explaining basic concepts of probability and disorder susceptibility. The nurse should ensure complete informed consent to facilitate decisions about genetic testing. The nurse should explain ethical and legal issues related to genetics as well. The nurse should never instruct the client on which decision to make and should let the client make the decision.

CHAPTER 11

Activity A

1. cortisol
2. Ambivalence
3. Oxytocin
4. placenta
5. estrogen

6. sacroiliac
7. hemorrhoids
8. progesterone
9. Colostrum
10. leukorrhea

Activity B

1. The skin change is known as linea nigra, which develops during pregnancy in the middle of the abdomen, extending from the umbilicus to the pubic area.
2. **a.** Good food sources of folic acid include dark green vegetables, such as broccoli, romaine lettuce, and spinach; baked beans; black-eyed peas; citrus fruits; peanuts; and liver.
   b. The FDA has advised pregnant women and nursing mothers to avoid eating shark, swordfish, king mackerel, and tilefish because they contain traces of mercury that may harm a developing fetus.

Activity C

1. e   **2.** a   **3.** c   **4.** d   **5.** b

Activity D

1.

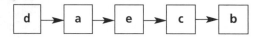

Activity E

1. Striae gravidarum, or stretch marks, are irregular reddish streaks that may appear on the abdomen, breasts, and buttocks in about half of pregnant women. Striae are most prominent by 6 to 7 months and occur in up to 90% of pregnant women. They are caused by reduced connective tissue strength resulting from elevated adrenal steroid levels and stretching of the structures secondary to growth. They are more common in younger women, women with larger infants, and women with higher body mass indices. Nonwhites and women with a history of breast or thigh striae or a family history of striae gravidarum are also at higher risk.
2. There is slight hypertrophy, or enlargement of the heart, during pregnancy to accommodate the increase in blood volume and cardiac output. The heart works harder and pumps more blood to supply the oxygen needs of the fetus as well as those of the mother. Both heart rate and venous return are increased in pregnancy, contributing to the increase in cardiac output seen throughout gestation.
3. Iron requirements during pregnancy increase because of the oxygen and nutrient demands of the growing fetus and the resulting increase in maternal blood volume. The fetal tissues take predominance over the mother's tissues with respect to use of iron stores. With the accelerated production of RBCs, iron is necessary for hemoglobin formation, the oxygen-carrying component of RBCs.

4. Pica is the compulsive ingestion of nonfood substances. The three main substances consumed by women with pica are soil or clay (geophagia), ice (pagophagia), and laundry starch (amylophagia). Nutritional implications of pica include iron-deficiency anemia, parasitic infection, and constipation.
5. Oxytocin is responsible for stimulating uterine contractions. After delivery, oxytocin secretion causes the myometrium to contract and helps constrict the uterine blood vessels, decreasing the amount of vaginal bleeding after delivery. Oxytocin is also responsible for milk ejection during breast-feeding. Stimulation of the breasts through sucking or touching stimulates the secretion of oxytocin from the posterior pituitary gland.
6. Varicose veins during pregnancy are the result of venous distention and instability, from poor circulation secondary to prolonged standing or sitting. Venous compression from the heavy gravid uterus places pressure on the pelvic veins, also preventing efficient venous return.

Activity F

1. **a.** The realization of a pregnancy can lead to fluctuating responses, possibly at opposite ends of the spectrum. For example, regardless of whether the pregnancy was planned, it is normal to be fearful and anxious of the implications. Your reaction may be influenced by several factors, including the way you were raised by your family, your current family situation, the quality of the relationship with the expectant father, and your hopes for the future. It is common for some women to express concern over the timing of the pregnancy, wishing that goals and life objectives had been met before becoming pregnant. Other women may question how a newborn or infant will affect their careers or their relationships with friends and family. These feelings can cause conflict and confusion about the impending pregnancy.

   Ambivalence, or having conflicting feelings at the same time, is a universal feeling and is considered normal when preparing for a lifestyle change and new role. Pregnant women commonly experience ambivalence during the first trimester. Usually ambivalence evolves into acceptance by the second trimester, when fetal movement is felt.
   b. A pregnant woman may withdraw and become increasingly preoccupied with herself and her fetus. As a result, participation with the outside world may be less, and she may appear passive to her family and friends. This introspective behavior is a normal psychological adaptation to motherhood for most women. Introversion seems to heighten during the first and third trimesters, when the woman's focus is on behaviors that will ensure a safe and healthy pregnancy outcome. Women may also feel disinterested in certain

activities because of nausea and fatigue experienced in the first trimester. Couples need to be aware of this behavior and be informed about measures to maintain and support the focus on the family.

c. During the second trimester, as the pregnancy progresses, the physical changes of the growing fetus, along with an enlarging abdomen and fetal movement, bring reality and validity to the pregnancy. The pregnant woman feels fetal movement and may hear the heartbeat. She may see the fetal image on an ultrasound screen and feel distinct parts, which allow her to identify the fetus as a separate individual. Many women will verbalize positive feelings of the pregnancy and will conceptualize the fetus. In addition, a reduction in physical discomfort will bring about an improvement in mood and physical well-being in the second trimester.

d. Frequently, pregnant women will start to cry without any apparent cause. Some feel as though they are riding an "emotional roller coaster." These extremes in emotion can make it difficult for partners and family members to communicate with the pregnant woman without placing blame on themselves for the woman's mood changes. Emotional lability is characteristic throughout most pregnancies. One moment a woman can feel great joy, and within a short time span feel shock and disbelief.

Activity G

1. Answer: b
RATIONALE: Absence of menstruation, or skipping a period, along with consistent nausea, fatigue, breast tenderness, and urinary frequency, are the presumptive signs of pregnancy. A positive home pregnancy test, abdominal enlargement, and softening of the cervix are the probable signs of pregnancy.

2. Answer: c
RATIONALE: During pregnancy, the vaginal secretions become more acidic, white, and thick. Most women experience an increase in a whitish vaginal discharge, called leukorrhea, during pregnancy. The nurse should inform the client that the vaginal discharge is normal except when it is accompanied by itching and irritation, possibly suggesting *Candida albicans* infection, a monilial vaginitis, which is a very common occurrence in this glycogen-rich environment. Monilial vaginitis is a benign fungal condition and is treated with local antifungal agents. The client need not refrain from sexual activity when there is an increase in a thick, whitish vaginal discharge.

3. Answer: a
RATIONALE: Estrogen aids in developing the ductal system of the breasts in preparation for lactation during pregnancy. Prolactin stimulates the glandular production of colostrum. During pregnancy, the ability of prolactin to produce milk is opposed by progesterone. Progesterone supports the endometrium of the uterus to provide an environment conducive to fetal survival. Oxytocin is responsible for uterine contractions, both before and after delivery. Oxytocin is also responsible for milk ejection during breastfeeding.

4. Answer: d
RATIONALE: The maternal emotional response experienced by the client is ambivalence. Ambivalence, or having conflicting feelings at the same time, is universal and is considered normal when preparing for a lifestyle change and new role. Pregnant women commonly experience ambivalence during the first trimester. The client is not experiencing introversion, acceptance, or mood swings. Introversion, or focusing on oneself, is common during the early part of pregnancy. The woman may withdraw and become increasingly preoccupied with herself and her fetus. Acceptance is the common maternal emotional response during the second trimester. As the pregnancy progresses, the physical changes of the growing fetus, along with an enlarging abdomen and fetal movement, bring reality and validity to the pregnancy. Although mood swings are common during pregnancy, this client is not experiencing mood swings.

5. Answer: a, c, & e
RATIONALE: Constipation during pregnancy is due to changes in the gastrointestinal system. Constipation can result from decreased activity level, use of iron supplements, intestinal displacement secondary to a growing uterus, slow transition time of food throughout the GI tract, a low-fiber diet, and reduced fluid intake. Increase in progesterone, not estrogen levels, causes constipation during pregnancy. Reduced stomach acidity does not cause constipation. Morning sickness has been linked to stomach acidity.

6. Answer: a, b, & d
RATIONALE: hCG levels in a normal pregnancy usually double every 48 to 72 hours, until they reach a peak at approximately 60 to 70 days after fertilization. This elevation of hCG corresponds to the morning sickness period of approximately 6 to 12 weeks during early pregnancy. Reduced stomach acidity and high levels of circulating estrogens are also believed to cause morning sickness. Elevation of hPL and RBC production do not cause morning sickness. hPL increases during the second half of pregnancy, and it helps in the preparation of mammary glands for lactation and is involved in the process of making glucose available for fetal growth by altering maternal carbohydrate, fat, and protein metabolism. The increase in RBCs is necessary to transport the additional oxygen required during pregnancy.

7. Answer: c
RATIONALE: Spontaneous, irregular, painless contractions, called Braxton Hicks contractions, begin during the first trimester. These contractions are

not the signs of preterm labor, infection of the GI tract, or acid indigestion. Acid indigestion causes heartburn. Acid indigestion or heartburn (pyrosis) is caused by regurgitation of the stomach contents into the upper esophagus and may be associated with the generalized relaxation of the entire digestive system.

8. **Answer: d**

   RATIONALE: The symptoms experienced by the client indicate supine hypotension syndrome. When the pregnant woman assumes a supine position, the expanding uterus exerts pressure on the inferior vena cava, causing a reduction in blood flow to the heart, most commonly during the third trimester. The nurse should place the client in the left lateral position to correct this syndrome and optimize cardiac output and uterine perfusion. Elevating the client's legs, placing the client in an orthopneic position, or keeping the head of the bed elevated will not help alleviate the client's condition.

9. **Answer: a**

   RATIONALE: The nurse should instruct the parents to provide constant reinforcement of love and care to reduce the sibling's fear of change and possible replacement by the new family member. The parents should neither avoid talking to the child about the new arrival nor pay less attention to the child. The nurse should urge parents to include siblings in this event and make them feel a part of the preparations for the new infant. The nurse should instruct the parents to continue to focus on the older sibling after the birth to reduce regressive or aggressive behavior that might manifest toward the newborn. The child is exhibiting sibling rivalry, which results from the child's fear of change in the security of his relationships with his parents. This behavior is common and does not require the intervention of a child psychologist.

10. **Answer: b**

    RATIONALE: Monilial vaginitis is a benign fungal condition that is uncomfortable for women; it can be transmitted from an infected mother to her newborn at birth. Neonates develop an oral infection known as thrush, which presents as white patches on the mucus membranes of the mouth. Although rubella, toxoplasmosis, and cytomegalovirus are infections transmitted to the newborn by the mother, this newborn is not experiencing any of these infections. Rubella causes fetal defects, known as congenital rubella syndrome; common defects of rubella are cataracts, deafness, congenital heart defects, cardiac disease, and mental retardation. Possible fetal effects due to toxoplasmosis include stillbirth, premature delivery, microcephaly, hydrocephaly, seizures, and mental retardation, whereas possible effects of cytomegalovirus infection include SGA, microcephaly, hydrocephaly, and mental retardation.

11. **Answer: a**

    RATIONALE: Between 38 and 40 weeks of gestation, the fundal height drops as the fetus begins to descend and engage into the pelvis. Because it pushes against the diaphragm, many women experience shortness of breath. By 40 weeks, the fetal head begins to descend and engage into the pelvis. Although breathing becomes easier because of this descent, the pressure on the urinary bladder now increases, and women experience urinary frequency. The fundus reaches its highest level at the xiphoid process at approximately 36, not 39, weeks. By 20 weeks' gestation, the fundus is at the level of the umbilicus and measures 20 cm. At between 6 and 8 weeks of gestation, the cervix begins to soften (Goodell's sign) and the lower uterine segment softens (Hegar's sign).

12. **Answer: c**

    RATIONALE: The skin and complexion of pregnant women undergo hyperpigmentation, primarily as a result of estrogen, progesterone, and melanocyte-stimulating hormone levels. The increased pigmentation that occurs on the breasts and genitalia also develops on the face to form the "mask of pregnancy," or facial melasma. This is a blotchy, brownish pigment that covers the forehead and cheeks in dark-haired women. The symptoms experienced by the client do not indicate linea nigra, striae gravidarum, or vascular spiders. The skin in the middle of the abdomen may develop a pigmented line called the linea nigra, which extends from the umbilicus to the pubic area. Striae gravidarum, or stretch marks, are irregular reddish streaks that appear on the abdomen, breasts, and buttocks in about 50% of pregnant women after month 5 of gestation. Vascular spiders appear as small, spider-like blood vessels in the skin and are usually found above the waist and on the neck, thorax, face, and arms.

13. **Answer: c**

    RATIONALE: During pregnancy, there is an increase in the client's blood components. These changes, coupled with venous stasis secondary to venous pooling, which occurs during late pregnancy after standing long periods of time (with the pressure exerted by the uterus on the large pelvic veins), contribute to slowed venous return, pooling, and dependent edema. These factors also increase the woman's risk for venous thrombosis. The symptoms experienced by the client do not indicate that she is at risk for hemorrhoids, embolism, or supine hypotension syndrome. Supine hypotension syndrome occurs when the uterus expands and exerts pressure on the inferior vena cava, which causes a reduction in blood flow to the heart. A client with supine hypotension syndrome experiences dizziness, clamminess, and a marked decrease in blood pressure.

14. Answer: a, c, & e

RATIONALE: Changes in the structures of the respiratory system take place to prepare the body for the enlarging uterus and increased lung volume. Increased vascularity of the respiratory tract is influenced by increased estrogen levels, leading to congestion. This congestion gives rise to nasal and sinus stuffiness and to epistaxis (nosebleed). As muscles and cartilage in the thoracic region relax, the chest broadens with a conversion from abdominal breathing to thoracic breathing. Persistent cough, Kussmaul's respirations, and dyspnea are not associated with the changes in the respiratory tract during pregnancy.

15 Answer: d

RATIONALE: During the second trimester, many women will verbalize positive feelings about the pregnancy and will conceptualize the fetus. The woman may accept her new body image and talk about the new life within her. Generating a discussion about the woman's feelings and offering support and validation at prenatal visits are important nursing interventions. The nurse should encourage the client in her first trimester to focus on herself, not on the fetus; this is not required when the client is in her second trimester. The client's feelings are normal for the second trimester of pregnancy; hence, it is not necessary either to inform the primary health care provider about the client's feelings or to tell the client that it is too early to conceptualize the fetus.

16. Answer: b

RATIONALE: The nurse should instruct the client to change sexual positions to increase comfort as the pregnancy progresses. Although the nurse should also encourage her to engage in alternative, non-coital modes of sexual expression, such as cuddling, caressing, and holding, the client need not restrict herself to such alternatives. It is not advisable to perform frequent douching, because this is believed to irritate the vaginal mucosa and predispose the client to infection. Using lubricants or performing stress-relieving and relaxation exercises will not alleviate discomfort during sexual activity.

17. Answer: b

RATIONALE: During the second trimester of pregnancy, partners go through acceptance of their role of breadwinner, caretaker, and support person. They come to accept the reality of the fetus when movement is felt, and they experience confusion when dealing with the woman's mood swings and introspection. During the first trimester, the expectant partner may experience couvade syndrome—a sympathetic response to the partner's pregnancy—and may also experience ambivalence with extremes of emotions. During the third trimester, the expectant partner prepares for the reality of the new role and negotiates what his or her role will be during the labor and birthing process.

CHAPTER 12

Activity A

1. doula
2. primipara
3. Fundal
4. Montgomery's
5. Chadwick's
6. Pica
7. Amniocentesis
8. liver
9. nonstress
10. Hemorrhoids

Activity B

1. **a.** The figure shows the procedure for amniocentesis. Amniocentesis involves a transabdominal perforation of the amniotic sac to obtain a sample of amniotic fluid for analysis.

   b. The fluid contains fetal cells that are examined to detect chromosomal abnormalities and several hereditary metabolic defects in the fetus before birth. Amniocentesis is also used to confirm a fetal abnormality when other screening tests detect a possible problem.

2. **a.** The figure shows a pregnant client using pillows for support in the side-lying position.

   b. Using pillows for support in the side-lying position relieves pressure on major blood vessels that supply oxygen and nutrients to the fetus when resting.

Activity C

1. d   2. e   3. a   4. b   5. c

Activity D

1.

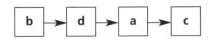

Activity E

1. The nurse should include the following key areas when providing preconception care:
   - Immunization status
   - Underlying medical conditions, such as cardiovascular or respiratory problems or genetic disorders
   - Reproductive health data such as pelvic examinations, use of contraceptives, and sexually transmitted infections (STIs)
   - Sexuality and sexual practices, such as safe sex practices and body image issues
   - Nutrition
   - Lifestyle practices, including occupation and recreational activities
   - Psychosocial issues such as levels of stress and exposure to abuse and violence
   - Medication and drug use, including use of tobacco, alcohol, over-the-counter and prescription medications, and illicit drugs

- Support system, including family, friends, and community

2. Nurses can enter into a collaborative partnership with a woman and her partner, enabling them to examine their own health and its influence on the health of their future baby. The nurse performs the following interventions as part of preconception care to ensure a positive impact on the pregnancy:
   - Stress the importance of taking folic acid to prevent neural tube defects
   - Urge the woman to achieve optimal weight before pregnancy
   - Ensure that the woman's immunizations are up to date
   - Address substance use issues, including smoking and taking drugs
   - Identify victims of violence and assist them in getting help
   - Manage chronic conditions such as diabetes and asthma
   - Educate the woman about environmental hazards, including metals and herbs
   - Offer genetic counseling to identify carriers
   - Suggest the availability of support systems, if needed

3. The assessments to be made by a nurse on a client's initial prenatal visit are as follows:
   - Screen for factors that place the client and her fetus at risk
   - Educate the client about changes that will affect her life

4. Counseling and educating the pregnant client and her partner are important to healthy outcomes for the mother and her infant. The role of a nurse in providing counseling and education to the client during a prenatal visit is as follows:
   - Provide anticipatory guidance
   - Make appropriate community referrals
   - Answer questions that the client and her partner may have regarding the pregnancy. It is important for the nurse to clarify all the misinformation or misconceptions in the minds of the client and her partner.

5. The nurse should perform the following assessments when conducting a chest examination of the client:
   - Auscultate heart sounds, noting any abnormalities
   - A soft systolic murmur caused by the increase in blood volume may be noted
   - Anticipate an increase in heart rate by 10 to 15 beats per minute secondary to increases in cardiac output and blood volume
   - Note adaptation of the body with peripheral dilatation
   - Auscultate the chest for breath sounds, which should be clear
   - Note symmetry of chest movement and thoracic breathing patterns

- Expect a slight increase in respiratory rate to accommodate the increase in tidal volume and oxygen consumption
- Inspect and palpate the breasts: increases in estrogen and progesterone and blood supply make the breasts feel full and more nodular, with increased sensitivity to touch
- Blood vessels become more visible, and there is an increase in breast size
- Striae gravidarum may be visible in women with large breasts
- Darker pigmentation of the nipple and areola is present, along with enlargement of Montgomery's glands
- Teach and reinforce breast self-examination

6. The nurse should perform the following assessments during a follow-up visit:
   - Weight and blood pressure, which are compared to baseline values
   - Urine testing for protein, glucose, ketones, and nitrites
   - Fundal height measurement to assess fetal growth
   - Assessment for quickening/fetal movement to determine well-being
   - Assessment of fetal heart rate (should be 120 to 160 bpm)
   - Answer questions
   - Provide anticipatory guidance and education
   - Review nutritional guidelines
   - Evaluate the client for compliance with prenatal vitamin therapy
   - Encourage the woman's partner to participate if possible

Activity F

1. a. The items in the checklist used by the nurse to ensure that the client is well prepared for the newborn's birth and homecoming are as follows:
   - Attend childbirth preparation classes and practice breathing techniques
   - Purchase an infant safety seat
   - Select a feeding method
   - Decide whether a boy will be circumcised
   - Select and arrange for a birth setting
   - Tour the birthing facility
   - Choose a family planning method to be used after the birth
   - Communicate needs and desires concerning pain management
   - Understand signs and symptoms of labor
   - Provide for care of other siblings during labor (when applicable)
   - Discuss the possibility of a cesarean birth
   - Prepare for the birthing facility when labor starts
   - Discuss possible names for the newborn
   - Know how to reach a health care professional when labor starts
   - Decide on a pediatrician

b. The nurse should perform the following interventions in preparing a client for breastfeeding:
- Encourage the client to attend a La Leche League class.
- Provide the client with sources of information about infant feeding.
- Suggest that the client read a good reference book about lactation.

c. The nurse should educate the pregnant client about the following advantages of breastfeeding:
- Human milk is digestible, is economical, and requires no preparation.
- Promotes bonding between mother and child
- Costs less than purchasing formula
- Suppresses ovulation
- Reduces the risk of ovarian cancer and premenopausal breast cancer
- Uses extra calories, which promotes weight loss gradually without dieting
- Releases oxytocin, which promotes rapid uterine involution with less bleeding
- Suckling helps in developing the muscles in the infant's jaw
- Improves absorption of lactose and minerals in the newborn
- Helps prevent infections in the baby
- Composition of breast milk adapts to meet the infant's changing needs
- Prevents constipation in the baby, with adequate intake
- Helps lessen chance that the baby will develop food allergies
- Reduces the incidence of otitis media and upper respiratory infections in the infant and the risk of adult obesity
- Makes the baby less prone to vomiting

Activity G

1. Answer: c
RATIONALE: When preparing the client for a physical examination, the nurse should instruct the client to empty her bladder; the nurse should then collect the urine sample so that it can be sent for laboratory tests to detect possibilities of a urinary tract infection. The client need not lie down, take deep breaths, or have the family present; however, it is important for the nurse to ensure that the client feels comfortable.

2. Answer: a
RATIONALE: To reduce the client's urinary frequency, the nurse should instruct the client to avoid consuming caffeinated drinks, since caffeine stimulates voiding patterns. The nurse instructs the client to drink fluids between meals rather than with meals, if the client complains of nausea and vomiting. The nurse instructs the client to avoid an empty stomach at all times, to prevent fatigue. The nurse also instructs the client to munch on dry crackers or toast early in the morning before arising if the client experiences nausea and vomiting; this would not help the client experiencing urinary frequency.

3. Answer: a, b, & c
RATIONALE: When documenting a comprehensive health history while caring for a client, it is important for the nurse to prepare a care plan that suits the client's lifestyle, to develop a trusting relationship with the client, and to prepare a plan of care for the pregnancy. The nurse does not need to assess the client's partner's sexual health during the history-taking process or urge the client to achieve an optimal body weight. Achieving optimal body weight before conception helps the client to achieve a positive impact on the pregnancy.

4. Answer: a, d, & e
RATIONALE: While conducting a physical examination of the head and neck, the nurse assesses for any previous injuries and sequelae, evaluates for limitations in range of motion, and palpates the thyroid gland for enlargement. The nurse should also assess for any edema of the nasal mucosa or hypertrophy of gingival tissue, as well as palpate for enlarged lymph nodes or swelling. The nurse need not check the client's eye movements; pregnancy does not affect the eye muscles. The nurse should check for levels of estrogen when examining the extremities of the client.

5. Answer: d
RATIONALE: In the 12th week of gestation, the nurse should palpate the fundus at the symphysis pubis. The nurse should palpate for the fundus below the ensiform cartilage when the client is in the 36th week of gestation; midway between symphysis and umbilicus in the 16th week of gestation; and at the umbilicus in the 20th week of gestation.

6. Answer: c
RATIONALE: While examining external genitalia, the nurse should assess for any infection due to hematomas, varicosities, inflammation, lesions, and discharge. The nurse assesses for a long, smooth, thick, and closed cervix when examining the internal genitalia. Other assessments when examining the internal genitalia include assessing for bluish coloration of cervix and vaginal mucosa and conducting a rectal examination to assess for lesions, masses, prolapse, or hemorrhoids.

7. Answer: b
RATIONALE: When assessing fetal well-being through abdominal ultrasonography, the nurse should instruct the client to refrain from emptying her bladder. The nurse must ensure that abdominal ultrasonography is conducted on a full bladder and should inform the client that she is likely to feel cold, not hot, initially in the test. The nurse should obtain the client's vital records and instruct the client to report the occurrence of fever when the client has to undergo amniocentesis, not ultrasonography.

8. **Answer: a**

   RATIONALE: The nurse should inform the client that sexual activity is permissible during pregnancy unless there is a history of incompetent cervix, vaginal bleeding, placenta previa, risk of preterm labor, multiple gestation, premature rupture of membranes, or presence of any infection. Anemia and facial and hand edema would be contraindications to exercising but not intercourse. Freedom from anxieties and worries contributes to adequate sleep promotion.

9. **Answer: a**

   RATIONALE: To help alleviate constipation, the nurse should instruct the client to ensure adequate hydration and bulk in the diet. The nurse should instruct the client to avoid spicy or greasy foods when a client complains of heartburn or indigestion. The nurse also should instruct the client to avoid lying down for two hours after meals if the client experiences heartburn or indigestion. The nurse should instruct the client to practice Kegel exercises when the client experiences urinary frequency.

10. **Answer: d**

    RATIONALE: To promote easy and safe travel for the client, the nurse should instruct the client to always wear a three-point seat belt to prevent ejection or serious injury from collision. The nurse should instruct the client to deactivate the air bag if possible. The nurse should instruct the client to apply a nonpadded shoulder strap properly, ensuring that it crosses between the breasts and over the upper abdomen, above the uterus. The nurse should instruct the client to use a lap belt that crosses over the pelvis below—not over—the uterus.

11. **Answer: b**

    RATIONALE: Nagele's rule can be used to establish the estimated date of birth. Using this rule, the nurse should subtract 3 months and then add 7 days to the first day of the last normal menstrual period. On the basis of Nagele's rule, the estimated date of birth (EDB) will be December 17, because the client started her last menstrual period on March 10. January 7, February 21, and January 30 are not the EDB according to Nagele's rule.

12. **Answer: a**

    RATIONALE: Pica is characterized by a craving for substances that have no nutritional value. Consumption of these substances can be dangerous to the client and her developing fetus. The nurse should monitor the client for iron-deficiency anemia as a manifestation of the client's compulsion to consume soil. Consumption of ice due to pica is likely to lead to tooth fractures. The nurse should monitor for inefficient protein metabolism if the client has been consuming laundry starch as a result of pica. The nurse should monitor for constipation in the client if she has been consuming clay.

13. **Answer: b, c, & e**

    RATIONALE: When caring for a pregnant client who follows a vegetarian diet, the nurse should monitor her for iron-deficiency anemia, decreased mineral absorption, and low gestational weight gain. Risk of epistaxis and increased risk of constipation are not reported to be associated with a vegetarian diet.

14. **Answer: a**

    RATIONALE: In a client's second trimester of pregnancy, the nurse should educate the client to look for vaginal bleeding as a danger sign of pregnancy needing immediate attention from the physician. Generally, painful urination, severe/persistent vomiting, and lower abdominal and shoulder pain are the danger signs that the client has to monitor for during the first trimester of pregnancy.

15. **Answer: c**

    RATIONALE: The nurse should instruct the client to serve the formula to her infant at room temperature. The nurse should instruct the client to follow the directions on the package when mixing the powder, because different formulas may have different instructions. The infant should be fed every 3 to 4 hours, not every 8 hours. The nurse should specifically instruct the client to avoid refrigerating the formula for subsequent feedings. Any leftover formula should be discarded.

16. **Answer: d**

    RATIONALE: According to the Lamaze method of preparing for labor and childbirth, the nurse must remain quiet during the client's period of imagery and focal point visualization to avoid breaking her concentration. The nurse should ensure deep abdominopelvic breathing by the client according to the Bradley method, along with ensuring the client's concentration on pleasurable sensations. The Bradley method emphasizes the pleasurable sensations of childbirth and involves teaching women to concentrate on these sensations when "turning on" to their own bodies. The nurse should ensure abdominal breathing during contractions when using the Dick-Read method.

17. **Answer: b**

    RATIONALE: To help the client alleviate varicosities of the legs, the nurse should instruct the client to refrain from crossing her legs when sitting for long periods. The nurse should instruct the client to avoid standing, not sitting, in one position for long periods. The nurse should instruct the client to wear support stockings to promote better circulation, though the client should stay away from constrictive stockings and socks. Applying heating pads on the extremities is not reported to alleviate varicosities of the legs.

18. **Answer: b, e, c, a, & d**

    RATIONALE: The client who is to undergo a nonstress test should have a meal before the procedure. The client is then placed in a lateral recumbent position to avoid supine hypotension syndrome. An external electronic fetal monitoring device is applied to her abdomen. The client is handed an "event marker" with a button that she pushes every time she perceives fetal movement. When the button is pushed, the fetal monitor strip is marked to identify that fetal movement has occurred.

CHAPTER 13

Activity A

1. gynecoid
2. effacement
3. sagittal
4. Zero
5. Lightening
6. contractions
7. decidua
8. passageway
9. nesting
10. molding

Activity B

1. **a.** The figure shows a frank breech presentation. In a frank breech, the buttocks present first, with both legs extended up toward the face.
   b. Breech presentations are associated with prematurity, placenta previa, multiparity, uterine abnormalities (fibroids), and some congenital anomalies such as hydrocephaly.
2. **a.** The figure shows a platypelloid, or flat, pelvis. This is the least common type of pelvic structure among men and women, with an approximate incidence of 5%.
   b. The pelvic cavity in a platypelloid (flat) pelvis is shallow but widens at the pelvic outlet, making it difficult for the fetus to descend through the midpelvis. It is not favorable for a vaginal birth unless the fetal head can pass through the inlet. Women with this type of pelvis usually require cesarean birth.

Activity C

1. a   2. b   3. e   4. d   5. c

Activity D

1.

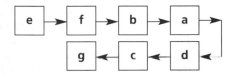

Activity E

1. Well-controlled research validates that nonmoving, back-lying positions during labor are not healthy. Despite this, most women lie flat on their backs. This position is preferred during labor mostly for the following reasons:

- Laboring women need to conserve their energy and not tire themselves
- Nurses can keep track of patients more easily if they are not ambulating
- The supine position facilitates vaginal examinations and external belt adjustment
- A bed is simply where one is usually supposed to be in a hospital setting
- Blind routine practice is convenient for the delivering health professional
- Laboring women are "connected to things" that impede movement

2. The nurse should encourage the pregnant client to adopt the upright or lateral position because such a position
- Reduces the duration of the second stage of labor
- Reduces the number of assisted deliveries (vacuum and forceps)
- Reduces episiotomies and perineal tears
- Contributes to fewer abnormal fetal heart rate patterns
- Increases comfort and reduces requests for pain medication
- Enhances a sense of control reported by mothers
- Alters the shape and size of the pelvis, which assists descent
- Assists gravity to move the fetus downward
- Reduces the length of labor

3. Maternal physiologic responses that occur as a woman progresses through childbirth include:
- Increase in heart rate, by 10 to 18 bpm
- Increase in cardiac output, by 10% to 15% during the first stage of labor and by 30% to 50% during the second stage of labor
- Increase in blood pressure, by 10 to 30 mm Hg during uterine contractions in all labor stages
- Increase in white blood cell count, to 25,000 to 30,000 cells/mm^3, perhaps as a result of tissue trauma
- Increase in respiratory rate, along with greater oxygen consumption, related to the increase in metabolism
- Decrease in gastric motility and food absorption, which may increase the risk of nausea and vomiting during the transition stage of labor
- Decrease in gastric emptying and gastric pH, which increases the risk of vomiting with aspiration
- Slight elevation in temperature, possibly as a result of an increase in muscle activity
- Muscular aches/cramps, as a result of a stressed musculoskeletal system involved in the labor process
- Increase in BMR and decrease in blood glucose levels because of the stress of labor

4. The factors that influence the ability of a woman to cope with labor stress include these:
- Previous birth experiences and their outcomes
- Current pregnancy experience
- Cultural considerations

- Involvement of support system
- Childbirth preparation
- Expectations of the birthing experience
- Anxiety level and fear of labor experience
- Feelings of loss of control
- Fatigue and weariness
- Anxiety levels

5. The signs of separation that indicate the placenta is ready to deliver are the following:
   - Uterus rises upward
   - Umbilical cord lengthens
   - Blood trickles suddenly from the vaginal opening
   - Uterus changes its shape to globular

6. The following factors ensure a positive birth experience for the pregnant client:
   - Clear information on procedures
   - Positive support; not being alone
   - Sense of mastery, self-confidence
   - Trust in staff caring for her
   - Positive reaction to the pregnancy
   - Personal control over breathing
   - Preparation for the childbirth experience

Activity F

1. **a.** Many women fear being sent home from the hospital with "false labor." All women feel anxious when they feel contractions, but they should be informed that labor can be a long process, especially if it is their first pregnancy. With first pregnancies, the cervix can take up to 20 hours to dilate completely. False labor is a condition occurring during the latter weeks of some pregnancies, in which irregular uterine contractions are felt but the cervix is not affected. In contrast, true labor is characterized by contractions occurring at regular intervals that increase in frequency, duration, and intensity. True labor contractions bring about progressive cervical dilation and effacement.

   b. The client should be instructed to stay home until contractions are 5 minutes apart, lasting 45–60 seconds and strong enough so that a conversation during one is not possible. She should be instructed to drink fluids and walk to assess if there is any change in her contractions. In true labor, contractions are regular, become closer together, and become stronger with time. The contraction starts in the back and radiates around toward the front of the abdomen.

   c. Changing positions and moving around during labor and birth do offer several benefits. Maternal position can influence pelvic size and contours. Changing position and walking affect the pelvis joints, and they facilitate fetal descent and rotation. Squatting enlarges the pelvic outlet by approximately 25%, whereas a kneeling position removes pressure on the maternal vena cava and assists to rotate the fetus in the posterior position.

The client should be encouraged to ask the nurse caring for her during labor if she can walk and have the nurse suggest positions to try.

   d. The second stage of labor begins with complete cervical dilation (10 cm) and effacement and ends with the birth of the newborn. Although the previous stage of labor primarily involved the thinning and opening of the cervix, this stage involves moving the fetus through the birth canal and out of the body. The cardinal movements of labor occur during the early phase of passive descent in the second stage of labor.

   Contractions occur every 2 to 3 minutes, last 60 to 90 seconds, and are described as strong by palpation. During this expulsive stage, the client may feel more in control and less irritable and agitated and be focused on the work of pushing. Traditionally, women have been taught to hold their breath to the count of 10, inhale again, push again, and repeat the process several times during a contraction. This sustained, strenuous style of pushing has been shown to lead to hemodynamic changes in the mother and interfere with oxygen exchange between the mother and the fetus. The newest protocol from the Association of Women's Health, Obstetric and Neonatal Nurses (AWHONN) recommends an open-glottis method in which air is released during pushing to prevent the buildup of intrathoracic pressure. During the second stage of labor, pushing can either follow a spontaneous urge or be directed by the nurse and/or health provider. The second stage of labor has two phases, related to the existence and quality of the maternal urge to push and to obstetric conditions related to fetal descent. The early phase of the second stage is called the pelvic phase, because it is during this phase that the fetal head is negotiating the pelvis, rotating, and advancing in descent. The later phase is called the perineal phase, because at this point the fetal head is lower in the pelvis and is distending the perineum. The occurrence of a strong urge to push characterizes the later phase of the second stage and has also been called the phase of active pushing. The perineum bulges and there is an increase in bloody show. The fetal head becomes apparent at the vaginal opening but disappears between contractions. When the top of the head no longer regresses between contractions, it is said to have crowned. The fetus rotates as it maneuvers out. The second stage commonly lasts up to 3 hours in a first labor.

Activity G

1. **Answer: b**

   RATIONALE: The nurse knows that the client is experiencing lightening. Lightening occurs when the fetal presenting part begins to descend into the maternal pelvis. The uterus lowers and moves into a more anterior position. The client may report increased respiratory capacity, decreased dyspnea, increased pelvic pressure, cramping, and low back pain. She also may note edema of the lower extremities as a result of the increased stasis of blood pooling, an increase in vaginal discharge, and more frequent urination. Some women report a sudden increase in energy before labor. This is sometimes referred to as nesting. Bloody show is a pink-tinged secretion that occurs when a small amount of blood released by cervical capillaries mixes with mucus. Braxton Hicks contractions are typically felt as a tightening or pulling sensation of the top of the uterus.

2. **Answer: a, b, & d**
RATIONALE: Upon seeing the increased prostaglandin levels, the nurse should assess for myometrial contractions, leading to a reduction in cervical resistance and subsequent softening and thinning of the cervix. The uterus of the client will appear boggy during the fourth stage of delivery, after the completion of pregnancy and birth. Hypotonic character of the bladder is also marked during the fourth stage of pregnancy, not when the prostaglandin levels rise, marking the onset of labor.

3. **Answer: a**
RATIONALE: Braxton Hicks contractions assist in labor by ripening and softening the cervix and moving the cervix from a posterior position to an anterior position. Prostaglandin levels increase late in pregnancy secondary to elevated estrogen levels; this is not due to the occurrence of Braxton Hicks contractions. Braxton Hicks contractions do not help in bringing about oxytocin sensitivity. Occurrence of lightening, not Braxton Hicks contractions, makes maternal breathing easier.

4. **Answer: c**
RATIONALE: The labor of a first-time-pregnant woman lasts longer because during the first pregnancy the cervix takes between 12 and 16 hours to dilate completely. The intensity of the Braxton Hicks contractions stays the same during the first and second pregnancies. Spontaneous rupture of membranes occurs before the onset of labor during each delivery, not only during the first delivery.

5. **Answer: d**
RATIONALE: The advantage of adopting a kneeling position during labor is that it helps to rotate the fetus in a posterior position. Facilitating vaginal examinations, facilitating external belt adjustment, and helping the woman in labor to save energy are advantages of the back-lying maternal position.

6. **Answer: a, b, & c**
RATIONALE: When caring for a client in labor, the nurse should monitor for an increase in the heart rate by 10 to 18 bpm, an increase in blood pressure by 10 to 30 mm Hg, and an increase in respiratory rate. During labor, the nurse should monitor for a slight elevation in body temperature as a result of

an increase in muscle activity. The nurse should also monitor for decreased gastric emptying and gastric pH, which increases the risk of vomiting with aspiration.

7. **Answer: d**
RATIONALE: When monitoring fetal responses in a client experiencing labor, the nurse should monitor for a decrease in circulation and perfusion to the fetus secondary to uterine contractions. The nurse should monitor for an increase, not a decrease, in arterial carbon dioxide pressure. The nurse should also monitor for a decrease, not an increase, in fetal breathing movements throughout labor. The nurse should monitor for a decrease in fetal oxygen pressure with a decrease in the partial pressure of oxygen.

8. **Answer: c**
RATIONALE: The nurse must massage the client's uterus briefly after placental expulsion to constrict the uterine blood vessels and minimize the possibility of hemorrhage. Massaging the client's uterus will not lessen the chances of conducting an episiotomy. In addition, an episiotomy, if required, is conducted in the second stage of labor, not the third. The client's uterus may appear boggy only in the fourth stage of labor—not in the third stage of labor. Ensuring that all sections of the placenta are present and that no piece is left attached to the uterine wall is confirmed through a placental examination after expulsion.

9. **Answer: d**
RATIONALE: The first stage of labor terminates with the dilation of the cervix diameter to 10 cm. Diffused abdominal cramping and rupturing of the fetal membrane occurs during the first stage of labor. Regular contractions occur at the beginning of the latent phase of the first stage; they do not mark the end of the first stage of labor.

10. **Answer: a, c, & e**
RATIONALE: The nurse knows that lower uterine segment distention, ^AQ4 stretching and tearing of the structures, and dilation of the cervix cause pain in the first stage. The fetus moves along the birth canal during the second stage of labor, when the client is more in control and less agitated. Spontaneous expulsion of the placenta occurs in the third stage of labor, not the first.

11. **Answer: b**
RATIONALE: The nurse, along with the physician, has to assess for fetal anomalies, which are usually associated with a shoulder presentation during a vaginal birth. The other conditions include placenta previa and multiple gestations. Uterine abnormalities, congenital anomalies, and prematurity are conditions associated with a breech presentation of the fetus during a vaginal birth.

12. **Answer: a, b, & c**
RATIONALE: To ensure a positive childbirth experience for the client, the nurse should provide the client clear information on procedures involved,

encourage the client to have a sense of mastery and self-control, and encourage the client to have a positive reaction to pregnancy. Instructing the client to spend some time alone is not an appropriate intervention; instead, the nurse should instruct the client to obtain positive support and avoid being alone. The client does not need to change the home environment; this does not ensure a positive childbirth experience.

13. **Answer: c**
RATIONALE: If the long axis of the fetus is perpendicular to that of the mother, then the client's fetus is in the transverse lie position. If the long axis of the fetus is parallel to that of the mother, the client's fetus is in the longitudinal lie position. The long axis of the fetus being at 45 or 60 degrees to that of the client does not indicate any specific position of the fetus.

14. **Answer: d**
RATIONALE: The pauses between contractions during labor are important because they allow the restoration of blood flow to the uterus and the placenta. Shortening of the upper uterine segment, reduction in length of the cervical canal, and effacement and dilation of the cervix are other processes that occur during uterine contractions.

15 **Answer: c**
RATIONALE: A shoulder presentation may be caused by anything that prevents the descent of the head or the breech into the lower pelvis. The condition that the nurse should try to observe during vaginal birth to identify a shoulder presentation is multiple gestations. The other conditions that should be observed are placenta previa and fetal anomalies. Multiparity, uterine abnormalities, and congenital anomalies are factors associated with breech presentations.

16. **Answer: a, c, & d**
RATIONALE: To provide comfort to the pregnant client, the nurse should make use of massage, hand holding, and acupressure to bring comfort to the pregnant client during labor. It is not advisable to provide chewing gum to a client in labor; it may cause accidental asphyxiation. Pain killers are not prescribed for a client experiencing labor.

CHAPTER 14

Activity A

1. Nonpharmacologic
2. hypoglycemia
3. fern
4. uteroplacental
5. ischial
6. uterine
7. tocotransducer
8. Artifact
9. parasympathetic
10. accelerations

Activity B

1. **a.** The FHR pattern shown in the image indicates late decelerations.
   b. Late decelerations are associated with uteroplacental insufficiency, which occurs when blood flow within the intervillous space is decreased to the extent that fetal hypoxia occurs. Conditions that may decrease uteroplacental perfusion with resultant decelerations include maternal hypotension, gestational hypertension, placental aging secondary to diabetes and postmaturity, hyperstimulation via oxytocin infusion, maternal smoking, anemia, and cardiac disease.

Activity C

1. c   **2.** b   **3.** a   **4.** d

Activity D

1.

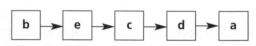

Activity E

1. The nurse should include biographical data such as the woman's name and age and the name of the delivering health care provider, prenatal record data, past health and family history, prenatal education, medications, risk factors, reason for admission, history of previous preterm births, allergies, the last time the client ate, method for infant feeding, name of birth attendant and pediatrician, and pain management plan.
2. The Apgar score assesses five parameters—heart rate (absent, slow, or fast), respiratory effort (absent, weak cry, or good strong yell), muscle tone (limp, or lively and active), response to irritation stimulus, and color—that evaluate a newborn's cardiorespiratory adaptation after birth.
3. The purpose of vaginal examination is to assess the amount of cervical dilation, the percentage of cervical effacement, and the fetal membrane status, and to gather information about presentation, position, station, degree of fetal head flexion, and presence of fetal skull swelling or molding.
4. Advantage: Electronic fetal monitoring produces a continuous record of the fetal heart rate, unlike intermittent auscultation, when gaps are likely. Disadvantage: Continuous monitoring can limit maternal movement and encourages her to lie in the supine position, which reduces placental perfusion.
5. The typical signs of the second stage of labor are as follows:
   • Increase in apprehension or irritability
   • Spontaneous rupture of membranes
   • Sudden appearance of sweat on upper lip
   • Increase in blood-tinged show
   • Low grunting sounds from the woman
   • Complaints of rectal and perineal pressure
   • Beginning of involuntary bearing-down efforts

6. Ideal positions for the second stage of labor are as follows:
- Lithotomy with feet up in stirrups: most convenient position for caregivers
- Semi-sitting with pillows underneath knees, arms, and back
- Lateral/side-lying with curved back and upper leg supported by partner
- Sitting on birthing stool: opens pelvis, enhances the pull of gravity, and helps with pushing
- Squatting/supported squatting: gives the woman a sense of control
- Kneeling with hands on bed and knees comfortably apart

Activity F

1. a. If there was no vaginal bleeding on admission, the nurse should perform a vaginal examination to assess cervical dilation, after which it is monitored periodically as necessary to identify progress.

b. The purpose of vaginal examination is to assess the amount of cervical dilation, the percentage of cervical effacement, and the fetal membrane status and to gather information about presentation, position, station, degree of fetal head flexion, and presence of fetal skull swelling or molding.

c. Procedure for conducting vaginal examination:
- Make the client comfortable
- Put on sterile gloves
- Use water as lubricant to check membrane status, if needed
- Use antiseptic solution to prevent infection if the membrane has ruptured
- Insert index and middle fingers into the vaginal introitus
- Palpate cervix to assess dilation, effacement, and position

Activity G

1. Answer: a
RATIONALE: When a nurse first comes in contact with a pregnant client during the admission assessment, it is important to first ascertain whether the woman is in true or false labor. Information regarding the number of pregnancies, addiction to drugs, or history of drug allergy is not important criteria for admitting the client.

2. Answer: a, c, & d
RATIONALE: When conducting an admission assessment on the phone for a pregnant client, the nurse needs to obtain information regarding the estimated due date, characteristics of contractions, and appearance of vaginal blood to evaluate the need to admit her. History of drug abuse or a drug allergy is usually recorded as part of the client's medical history.

3. Answer: b
RATIONALE: When a pregnant client is in the active phase of labor, the nurse should monitor the vital signs every 30 minutes. The nurse should monitor the vital signs every 30–60 minutes if the client is in the latent phase of labor and every 15–30 minutes during the transition phase of labor. Temperature is monitored every 4 hours in the active phase of labor.

4. Answer: a
RATIONALE: In a cephalic presentation, the FHR is best heard in the lower quadrant of the maternal abdomen. In a breech presentation, it is heard at or above the level of the maternal umbilicus.

5. Answer: c
RATIONALE: Fetal pulse oximetry measures fetal oxygen saturation directly and in real time. It is used with electronic fetal monitoring as an adjunct method of assessment when the FHR pattern is nonreassuring or inconclusive. Fetal scalp blood is obtained to measure the pH. The fetal position and weight can be determined through ultrasonography or abdominal palpation.

6. Answer: a
RATIONALE: Increased sedation is an adverse effect of lorazepam. Diazepam and midazolam cause central nervous system depression for both the woman and the newborn. Opioids are associated with newborn respiratory depression and decreased alertness.

7. Answer: d
RATIONALE: General anesthesia is administered in emergency cesarean births. Local anesthetic is injected into the superficial perineal nerves to numb the perineal area generally before an episiotomy. Although an epidural block is used in cesarean births, it is contraindicated in clients with spinal injury. Regional anesthesia is contraindicated in cesarean births.

8. Answer: b
RATIONALE: During the latent phase of labor, the nurse should monitor the FHR every hour. FHR should be monitored every 30 minutes in the active phase and every 15–30 minutes in the transition phase of labor. Continuous monitoring is done when an electronic fetal monitor is used.

9. Answer: b
RATIONALE: If vaginal bleeding is absent during admission assessment, the nurse should perform vaginal examination to assess the amount of cervical dilation. Hydration status is monitored as part of the physical examination. A urine specimen is obtained for urinalysis to obtain a baseline. Vital signs are monitored frequently throughout the maternal assessment.

10. Answer: c
RATIONALE: The nitrazine tape shows a pH between 5 and 6, which indicates an acidic environment with the presence of vaginal fluid and less blood. If the membranes had ruptured, amniotic fluid was present, or there was excess blood, the nitrazine test tape would have indicated an alkaline environment.

11. **Answer: a, b, & e**
RATIONALE: The nurse should assess the frequency of contractions, intensity of contractions, and uterine resting tone to monitor uterine contractions. Monitoring changes in temperature and blood pressure is part of the general physical examination and does not help to monitor uterine contraction.

12. **Answer: a, b, & c**
RATIONALE: Leopold's maneuvers help the nurse to determine the presentation, position, and lie of the fetus. The approximate weight and size of the fetus can be determined with ultrasound sonography or abdominal palpation.

13. **Answer: a, c, & d**
RATIONALE: The nurse should turn the client on her left side to increase placental perfusion, administer oxygen by mask to increase fetal oxygenation, and assess the client for any underlying contributing causes. The client's questions should not be ignored; instead, the client should be reassured that interventions are to effect FHR pattern change. A reduced IV rate would decrease intravascular volume, affecting the FHR further.

14. **Answer: c**
RATIONALE: The client should be administered oxygen by mask, because the nonreassuring FHR pattern could be due to inadequate oxygen reserves in the fetus. Because the client is in preterm labor, it is not advisable to apply vibroacoustic stimulation, tactile stimulation, or fetal scalp stimulation.

15. **Answer: a**
RATIONALE: The nurse must monitor for respiratory depression. Accidental intrathecal blockade, inadequate or failed block, and postdural puncture headache are possible complications associated with combined spinal-epidural analgesia.

16. **Answer: b**
RATIONALE: The nurse should provide supplemental oxygen if a client who has been administered combined spinal-epidural analgesia exhibits signs of hypotension and associated FHR changes. The client should be assisted to a semi-Fowler's position; the client should not be kept in a supine position or be turned on her left side. Discontinuing IV fluid will cause dehydration.

17. **Answer: b**
RATIONALE: The nurse should monitor the client for uterine relaxation. Pruritus, inadequate or failed block, and maternal hypotension are associated with combined spinal-epidural analgesia.

18. **Answer: a**
RATIONALE: The recommendation for initiating hydrotherapy is that women be in active labor (>5 cm dilated), to prevent the slowing of labor contractions secondary to muscular relaxation. Women are encouraged to stay in the bath or shower as long as they feel they are comfortable. The water temperature should not exceed body temperature. The woman's membranes can be intact or ruptured.

19. **Answer: b**
RATIONALE: For slow-paced breathing, the nurse should instruct the woman to inhale slowly through her nose and exhale through pursed lips. In shallow or modified-pace breathing, the woman should inhale and exhale through her mouth at a rate of 4 breaths every 5 seconds. In pattern-paced breathing, the breathing is punctuated every few breaths by a forceful exhalation through pursed lips. Holding the breath for 5 seconds after every three breaths is not recommended in any of the three levels of patterned breathing.

20. **Answer: a, b, & d**
RATIONALE: The nurse should check for any abnormality of the spine, hypovolemia, or coagulation defects in the client. An epidural is contraindicated in women with these conditions. Varicose veins and skin rashes or bruises are not contraindications for an epidural block. They are contraindications for massage used for pain relief during labor.

CHAPTER 15

Activity A
1. pelvis
2. subinvolution
3. Afterpains
4. engorgement
5. uterus
6. Oxytocin
7. nonlactating
8. Lactation
9. Prolactin
10. diaphoresis

Activity B
1. d   2. e   3. a   4. b   5. c

Activity C
1.

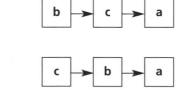

2.

Activity D
1. The timing of the first menses and ovulation after birth differs considerably in lactating and nonlactating women. In nonlactating women, menstruation resumes 7 to 9 weeks after giving birth; the first cycle is anovulatory. In lactating women, the return of menses depends on the frequency and duration of breastfeeding. It usually resumes anytime from 2 to 18 months after childbirth, and the first postpartum menses is usually heavier and frequently

anovulatory. However, ovulation may occur before menstruation, so breastfeeding is not a reliable method of contraception.

2. Afterpains are more acute in multiparous women secondary to repeated stretching of the uterine muscles, which reduces muscle tone, allowing for alternate uterine contraction and relaxation.

3. Factors that facilitate uterine involution are
   • Complete expulsion of amniotic membranes and placenta at birth
   • Complication-free labor and birth process
   • Breastfeeding
   • Ambulation

4. Factors that inhibit involution include
   • Prolonged labor and difficult birth
   • Incomplete expulsion of amniotic membranes and placenta
   • Uterine infection
   • Overdistention of uterine muscles due to
     a. Multiple gestation, hydramnios, or large singleton fetus
     b. Full bladder, which displaces uterus and interferes with contractions
     c. Anesthesia, which relaxes uterine muscles
     d. Close childbirth spacing, leading to frequent and repeated distention and thus decreasing uterine tone and causing muscular relaxation

5. Women who have had cesarean births tend to have less flow because the uterine debris is removed manually with delivery of the placenta.

6. Afterpains are usually stronger during breastfeeding because oxytocin released by the sucking reflex strengthens uterine contractions. Mild analgesics can be used to reduce this discomfort.

Activity E

1. a. The nurse should suggest the following measures to resolve engorgement in the client who is breastfeeding:
   Empty the breasts frequently to minimize discomfort and resolve engorgement.
   Stand in a warm shower or apply warm compresses to the breasts to provide some relief.
   b. The nurse should suggest the following relief measures for the client with non-breastfeeding engorgement:
   • Wear a tight, supportive bra 24 hours daily.
   • Apply ice to the breasts for approximately 15 to 20 minutes every other hour.
   • Do not stimulate the breasts by squeezing or manually expressing milk from the nipples.
   • Avoid exposing the breasts to warmth.

Activity F

1. **Answer: a, c, & d**
   RATIONALE: Involution involves three retrogressive processes. The first of these is contraction of muscle fibers, which serves to reduce those previously stretched during pregnancy. Next, catabolism reduces enlarged, individual myometrial cells.

Finally, there is regeneration of uterine epithelium from the lower layer of the decidua after the upper layers have been sloughed off and shed during lochia. The breasts do not return to their prepregnancy size as the uterus does. Urinary retention inhibits uterine involution.

2. **Answer: d**
   RATIONALE: Displacement of the uterus from the midline to the right and frequent voiding of small amounts suggests urinary retention with overflow. Catheterization may be necessary to empty the bladder to restore tone. A warm shower and warm compresses are recommended for clients with breastfeeding engorgement. Good body mechanics are recommended to prevent lower back and joint pains.

3. **Answer: b, c, & d**
   RATIONALE: The nurse should tell the client to use warm sitz baths, witch hazel pads, and anesthetic sprays to provide local comfort. Using good body mechanics and maintaining a correct position are important to prevent lower back pain and injury to the joints.

4. **Answer: a**
   RATIONALE: The nurse should recommend that the client practice Kegel exercises to improve pelvic floor tone, strengthen the perineal muscles, and promote healing. Witch hazel pads and sitz baths are useful in promoting local comfort in a client who had an episiotomy during the birth. Good body mechanics help to prevent lower back pain and injury to the joints.

5. **Answer: a, b, & d**
   RATIONALE: Many women have difficulty with feeling the sensation to void after giving birth if they have received an anesthetic block during labor, which inhibits neural functioning of the bladder. This client will be at risk for incomplete emptying, bladder distention, difficulty voiding, and urinary retention. Ambulation difficulty and perineal lacerations are due to episiotomy.

6. **Answer: c**
   RATIONALE: Postpartum diuresis is due to the buildup and retention of extra fluids during pregnancy. Bruising and swelling of the perineum, swelling of tissues surrounding the urinary meatus, and decreased bladder tone due to anesthesia cause urinary retention.

7. **Answer: b**
   RATIONALE: The nurse should recommend that clients maintain correct position and good body mechanics to prevent pain in the lower back, hips, and joints. Anesthetic sprays are used to provide local comfort for clients with a bruised or swollen perineum. Kegel exercises are recommended to promote pelvic floor tone. Application of ice is suggested to help relieve breast engorgement in non-breastfeeding clients.

8. **Answer: a**
RATIONALE: The nurse should suggest that the father care for the newborn by holding and talking to the child. Reading up on parental care and speaking to his friends or the physician will not help the father resolve his fears about caring for the child.

9. **Answer: c**
RATIONALE: The nurse should encourage the client to change her gown to prevent chilling and reassure the client that it is normal to have postpartal diaphoresis. The use of good body mechanics is recommended to prevent lower back and joint injuries. Sitz baths are encouraged to promote local comfort in clients who had an episiotomy during the birth. Kegel exercises are recommended to promote pelvic floor tone.

10. **Answer: c**
RATIONALE: The nurse should tell the client that poor perineal muscular tone may cause urinary incontinence later in life. Kegel exercises are important to improve perineal muscular tone. Pain in the joints and lower back is due to improper body position. Postpartum diuresis is observed in the first week after birth.

11. **Answer: c**
RATIONALE: The nurse should tell the client to frequently empty the breasts to improve milk supply. Encouraging cold baths and applying ice on the breasts are recommended to relieve engorgement in non-breastfeeding clients. Kegel exercises are encouraged to promote pelvic floor tone.

12. **Answer: a**
RATIONALE: The nurse should explain to the client that lochia rubra is a deep red mixture of mucus, tissue debris, and blood. Discharge consisting of leukocytes, decidual tissue, RBCs, and serous fluid is called lochia serosa. Discharge consisting of only RBCs and leukocytes is blood. Discharge consisting of leukocytes and decidual tissue is called lochia alba.

13. **Answer: d**
RATIONALE: The nurse should explain to the client that the afterpains are due to oxytocin released by the sucking reflex, which strengthens uterine contractions. Prolactin, estrogen, and progesterone cause synthesis and secretion of colostrum.

CHAPTER 16

Activity A
1. peribottle
2. mastitis
3. hypertension
4. Pain
5. Orthostatic
6. fundus
7. cesarean

8. Reciprocity
9. Commitment
10. colostrum

Activity B
1. c   **2.** a   **3.** d   **4.** b

Activity C
1. Postpartum assessment of the mother typically includes vital signs, pain level, and a systematic head-to-toe review of the body systems: breasts, uterus, bladder, bowels, lochia, episiotomy/perineum, extremities, and emotional status.

2. The new mother might ignore her own needs for health and nutrition. She should be encouraged to take good care of herself and eat a healthy diet so that the nutrients lost during pregnancy can be replaced and she can return to a healthy weight. The nurse should provide nutritional recommendations, such as
   • Eating a wide variety of foods with high nutrient density
   • Using foods and recipes that require little or no preparation
   • Avoiding high-fat, fast foods and fad weight-reduction diets
   • Drinking plenty of fluids
   • Avoiding harmful substances such as alcohol, tobacco, and drugs
   • Avoiding excessive intake of fat, salt, sugar, and caffeine
   • Eating the recommended daily servings from each food group

3. The physical stress of pregnancy and birth, the required care-giving tasks associated with a newborn, meeting the needs of other family members, and fatigue can cause the postpartum period to be quite stressful for the mother.

4. Postpartum danger signs include
   • Fever more than 38°C (100.4°F) after the first 24 hours following birth
   • Foul-smelling lochia or an unexpected change in color or amount
   • Visual changes, such as blurred vision or spots, or headaches
   • Calf pain experienced with dorsiflexion of the foot
   • Swelling, redness, or discharge at the episiotomy site
   • Dysuria, burning, or incomplete emptying of the bladder
   • Shortness of breath or difficulty breathing
   • Depression or extreme mood swings

5. The nurse should model behavior to family members as follows:
   • Holding the newborn close and speaking positively
   • Referring to the newborn by name in front of the parents
   • Speaking directly to the newborn in a calm voice

- Encouraging both parents to pick up and hold the newborn
- Monitoring newborn's response to parental stimulation
- Pointing out positive physical features of the newborn

6. The nurse should suggest the following to the family to avoid sibling rivalry:
   - Expect and tolerate some regression
   - Discuss the new infant during relaxed family times
   - Teach safe handling of the newborn with a doll
   - Encourage older children to verbalize emotions about the newborn
   - Move the sibling from the crib to a youth bed months in advance of the birth of the newborn

Activity D

1. **a.** The nurse should perform the following assessments in a client intending to breastfeed her baby:
   - Inspect the breasts for size, contour, asymmetry, engorgement, or areas of erythema.
   - Check the nipples for cracks, redness, fissures, or bleeding.
   - Palpate the breasts to ascertain if they are soft, filling, or engorged, and document findings.
   - Palpate the breasts for any nodules, masses, or areas of warmth, which may indicate a plugged duct that may progress to mastitis if not treated promptly.
   - Describe and document any discharge from the nipple that is not creamy yellow or bluish white.

   b. The client is encouraged to offer frequent feedings, at least every 2 to 3 hours, using manual expression just before feeding to soften the breast so the newborn can latch on more effectively. The client should be told to allow the newborn to feed on the first breast until it softens before switching to the other side.

Activity E

1. **Answer: b**
   RATIONALE: Postpartum assessment typically is performed every 15 minutes for the first hour. After the second hour, assessment is performed every 30 minutes. The client has to be monitored closely during the first hour after delivery; assessment frequencies of 45 minutes or 60 minutes are too long.

2. **Answer: c**
   RATIONALE: Tachycardia in the postpartum woman can suggest anxiety, excitement, fatigue, pain, excessive blood loss, infection, or underlying cardiac problems. Pulmonary edema, atelectasis, and pulmonary embolism are associated with out–of–normal-range changes in respiratory rate.

3. **Answer: d**
   RATIONALE: A boggy or relaxed uterus is a sign of uterine atony. This can be the result of bladder distention, which displaces the uterus upward and to the right, or retained placental fragments. Foul-smelling urine and purulent drainage are signs of infections but are not related to uterine atony. The firm fundus is normal and not a sign of uterine atony.

4. **Answer: b**
   RATIONALE: "Scant" would describe a one- to two-inch lochia stain on the perineal pad, or an approximate 10-mL loss. "Light" or "small" would describe an approximate four-inch stain, or a 10- to 25-mL loss. "Moderate" lochia would describe a four- to six- inch stain, with an estimated loss of 25 to 50 mL. A large or heavy lochia loss would describe pad saturation within an hour after changing it.

5. **Answer: d**
   RATIONALE: The nurse should classify the laceration as fourth-degree, because it continues through the anterior rectal wall. First-degree laceration involves only skin and superficial structures above muscle; second-degree laceration extends through perineal muscles; and third-degree laceration extends through the anal sphincter muscle but not through the anterior rectal wall.

6. **Answer: c**
   RATIONALE: The nurse should ensure that the ice pack is changed frequently to promote good hygiene and to allow for periodic assessments. Ice packs are wrapped in a disposable covering or clean washcloth and then applied to the perineal area, not directly. The nurse should apply the ice pack for 20 minutes, not 40 minutes. Ice packs should be used for the first 24 hours, not for a week after delivery.

7. **Answer: d**
   RATIONALE: Routine exercise should be resumed gradually, beginning with Kegel exercises on the first postpartum day. The client should be allowed to perform abdominal, buttock, and thigh-toning exercises only during the second week after delivery and not earlier.

8. **Answer: a**
   RATIONALE: The nurse should reassure the mother that some newborns "latch on and catch on" right away, and some newborns take more time and patience; this information will help to reduce the feelings of frustration and uncertainty about their ability to breastfeed. The nurse should also explain that breastfeeding is a learned skill for both parties. It would not be correct to say that breastfeeding is a mechanical procedure. In fact, the nurse should encourage the mother to cuddle and caress the infant while feeding. The nurse should allow sufficient time to the mother and child to enjoy each other in an unhurried atmosphere. The nurse should teach the mother to burp the infant frequently. Different positions, such as cradle and football holds and side-lying positions, should be shown to the mother.

9. **Answer: c**
   RATIONALE: The nurse should observe positioning and latching-on technique while breastfeeding so that she may offer suggestions based on observation to correct positioning/latching. This will help minimize trauma to the breast. The client should use only water, not soap, to clean the nipples to prevent dryness. Breast pads with plastic liners should be avoided. Leaving the nursing bra flaps down after feeding allows nipples to air dry.

10. **Answer: b**
    RATIONALE: The nurse should inform the client that intercourse can be resumed if bright-red bleeding stops. Use of water-based gel lubricants can be helpful and should not be avoided. Pelvic floor exercises may enhance sensation and should not be avoided. Barrier methods such as a condom with spermicidal gel or foam should be used instead of oral contraceptives.

11. **Answer: c**
    RATIONALE: The nurse should ensure that the follow-up appointment is fixed for within 2 weeks after hospital discharge. One week after hospital discharge is too early for a follow-up visit, whereas 3 weeks after discharge is too long because the client can develop complications that would go undiagnosed. For clients with an uncomplicated vaginal birth, an office visit is usually scheduled for between 4 and 6 weeks after childbirth.

12. **Answer: a**
    RATIONALE: Mothers who are Rh-negative and have given birth to an infant who is Rh-positive should receive an injection of Rh immunoglobulin within 72 hours after birth; this prevents a sensitization reaction to Rh-positive blood cells received during the birthing process. It may be too late to administer Rh immunoglobulin after 72 hours.

13. **Answer: a, b, & e**
    RATIONALE: Engorged breasts are hard, tender, and taut, and the nurse should assess for these signs. Improper positioning of the infant on the breast, not engorged breasts, results in cracked, blistered, fissured, bruised, or bleeding nipples in the breastfeeding woman.

14. **Answer: b, d, & e**
    RATIONALE: Finding active bowel sounds, verification of passing gas, and a nondistended abdomen are normal assessment results. The abdomen should be nontender and soft, not tender. Abdominal pain is not a normal assessment finding and should be immediately looked into.

15. **Answer: b, c, & e**
    RATIONALE: The nurse should show mothers how to initiate breastfeeding within 30 minutes of birth. To ensure bonding, place the baby in uninterrupted skin-to-skin contact with the mother. Breastfeeding on demand should be encouraged. Pacifiers should not be used because they do not help fulfill nutritional requirements.

The nurse should also ensure that no food or drink other than breast milk is given to newborns.

CHAPTER 17

Activity A
1. Habituation
2. reflex
3. acquired
4. Meconium
5. intestinal
6. amniotic
7. Jaundice
8. hemolysis
9. hemoglobin
10. hypothalamus

Activity B
1. d   **2.** a   **3.** c   **4.** b

Activity C
1. The newborn's response to auditory and visual stimuli is demonstrated by the following:
   - Moving the head and eyes to focus on stimulus
   - Staring at the object intently
   - Using sensory capacity to become familiar with people and objects
2. The expected neurobehavioral responses of the newborn include
   - Orientation
   - Habituation
   - Motor maturity
   - Self-quieting ability
   - Social behaviors
3. The following events must occur before the newborn's lungs can maintain respiratory function:
   - Initiation of respiratory movement
   - Expansion of the lungs
   - Establishment of functional residual capacity (ability to retain some air in the lungs on expiration)
   - Increased pulmonary blood flow
   - Redistribution of cardiac output
4. The amniotic fluid is removed from the lungs of a newborn by the following actions:
   - The passage through the birth canal squeezes the thorax, which helps eliminate the fluids in the lungs
   - The action of the pulmonary capillaries and lymphatics removes the remaining fluid
5. The nurse should look for the following signs of abnormality in the newborn's respiration:
   - Labored respiratory effort
   - Respiratory rate less than 30 breaths per minute or greater than 60 breaths per minute
   - Asymmetric chest movements
   - Periodic breathing
   - Apneic periods lasting more than 15 seconds with cyanosis and heart rate changes

6. The nursing interventions that may help minimize regurgitation are
   - Avoiding overfeeding
   - Stimulating frequent burping

Activity D

1. a. Normal factors that increase the heart rate and blood pressure in a newborn are
      - Wakefulness
      - Movement
      - Crying
   b. Normal factors affecting the hematologic values of a newborn are
      - Site of the blood sampling
      - Placental transfusion
      - Gestational age
   c. The benefits of delayed cord clamping after birth are
      - Improved cardiopulmonary adaptation and oxygen transport
      - Prevention of anemia
      - Increased blood pressures and RBC flow

Activity E

1. **Answer: b**
   RATIONALE: The nurse should instruct the mother to keep the newborn wrapped in a blanket, with a cap on its head. This ensures that the newborn is kept warm and helps prevent cold stress. Allowing cool air to circulate over the newborn's body leads to heat loss and is not desirable. Holding the newborn close to the body after taking a shower is not recommended, as the mother's body temperature will be lower than normal after a shower. The nurse need not instruct the client to refrain from using clothing and blankets in the crib. Using clothing and blankets in the crib is actually an effective means of reducing the newborn's exposed surface area and providing external insulation.

2. **Answer: a**
   RATIONALE: Breast milk is a major source of IgA, so breastfeeding is believed to have significant immunologic advantages over formula feeding. The newborn does not depend on IgD and IgE for defense mechanisms. IgM is found in blood and lymph fluid.

3. **Answer: a, c, & d**
   RATIONALE: Limited sweating ability, a crib that is too warm or one that is placed too close to a sunny window, and limited insulation are factors that predispose a newborn to overheating. The immaturity of the newborn's central nervous system makes it difficult to create and maintain balance between heat production, heat gain, and heat loss. Underdeveloped lungs do not increase the risk of overheating. Lack of brown fat will make the infant feel cold, because he or she will not have enough fat stores to burn in response to cold; it does not however, increase the risk of overheating.

4. **Answer: c**
   RATIONALE: The nurse should look for signs of lethargy and hypotonia in the newborn in order to confirm the occurrence of cold stress. Cold stress does not lead to any color change in the newborn's skin or urine. Cold stress leads to a decrease, not increase, in the newborn's body temperature.

5. **Answer: b**
   RATIONALE: Risk factors for the development of jaundice include drugs such as oxytocin, diazepam, and sulfisoxazole/erythromycin. Breastfeeding, not formula feeding, and male gender are other risk factors. Administering hepatitis A vaccine does not increase the risk of jaundice.

6. **Answer: d**
   RATIONALE: The possibility of fluid overload is increased and must be considered by a nurse when administering IV therapy to a newborn. IV therapy does not significantly increase heart rate or change blood pressure.

7. **Answer: b**
   RATIONALE: The nurse should tell the client not to worry, because it is perfectly normal for the stools of a formula-fed newborn to be greenish, loose, pasty, or formed in consistency, with an unpleasant odor. There is no need to administer vitamin K supplements, increase the newborn's fluid intake, or switch from formula to breast milk.

8. **Answer: b**
   RATIONALE: The ideal caloric intake for a term newborn to regain weight lost in the first week is 108 kcal/kg/day. Eighty kcal/kg/day is too little to meet the newborn's requirements, and 150 or 200 kcal/kg/day will be greater than the newborn's requirements.

9. **Answer: a**
   RATIONALE: Preterm newborns are at a greater risk for cold stress than term or post-term newborns. Formula-fed newborns and larger-than-average newborns are not at a greater risk for cold stress than preterm newborns.

10. **Answer: a**
    RATIONALE: The hand-to-mouth movement of the baby indicates the self-quieting ability of a newborn. Movement of the head and eyes, movements of the legs, and hyperactivity do not indicate the self-quieting ability of a newborn.

11. **Answer: c**
    RATIONALE: Typically, a newborn's blood glucose levels are assessed with use of a heel stick sample of blood on admission to the nursery, not 5 or 24 hours after admission to the nursery. It is also not necessary or even reasonable to check the glucose level only after the newborn has been fed.

12. **Answer: a**
    RATIONALE: The nurse should promote early breast-feeding to provide fuels for nonshivering

thermogenesis. The nurse can bathe the newborn if he or she is medically stable. The nurse can also use a radiant heat source while bathing the newborn to maintain the temperature. Skin-to-skin contact with the mother should be encouraged, not discouraged, if the newborn is stable. The infant transporter should be kept fully charged and heated at all times.

13. Answer: c

RATIONALE: The nurse should place the temperature probe over the newborn's liver. Skin temperature probes should not be placed over a bony area like the forehead, or an area with brown fat such as the buttocks. The newborn should be in a supine or side-lying position.

14. Answer: a

RATIONALE: The nurse should monitor for yellow skin or mucous membranes in an infant at risk for developing jaundice. Pinkish appearance of the tongue and bluish skin discoloration are not consequences of increased bilirubin levels. A heart rate of 120 bpm is also normal for an infant.

15. Answer: d

RATIONALE: The stools of a breastfed newborn are yellowish gold in color. They are not firm in shape or solid. The smell is usually sour. A formula-fed infant's stools are formed in consistency, while a breastfed infant's stools are stringy to pasty in consistency.

CHAPTER 18

Activity A

1. Apgar
2. Lanugo
3. Postmature
4. large
5. prothrombin
6. acrocyanosis
7. Milia
8. Harlequin
9. anterior
10. Cephalhematoma

Activity B

1. The figure shows common skin variations found in newborns:
   - A. Stork bite
   - B. Milia
   - C. Mongolian spots
   - D. Erythema toxicum
   - E. Nevus flammeus (port-wine stain)
   - F. Strawberry hemangioma
2. The figure depicts molding in a newborn's head. Molding is the elongated shaping of the fetal head to accommodate passage through the birth canal.

Activity C

1. b   **2.** a   **3.** c   **4.** d

Activity D

1.

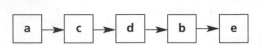

Activity E

1. The football hold is achieved by holding the infant's back and shoulders in the palm of the mother's hand and tucking the infant under the mother's arm. The infant's ear, shoulder, and hip should be in a straight line. The mother's hand should support the breast and bring it to the infant's lips to latch on until the infant begins to nurse. This position allows the mother to see the infant's mouth as she guides her infant to the nipple. Mothers who have had a cesarean birth can avoid pressure on the incision lines by adopting the football hold position for breastfeeding.

2. Colostrum is a thick, yellowish substance secreted during the first few days after birth. It is high in protein, minerals, and fat-soluble vitamins. It is rich in immunoglobulins (e.g., IgA), which help protect the newborn's GI tract against infections. It is a natural laxative to help rid the intestinal tract of meconium quickly.

3. Fiber optic pads (Biliblanket or Bilivest) are used for treatment of physiologic jaundice and can be wrapped around newborns or newborns can lie upon them. These pads consist of a light that is delivered from a tungsten–halogen bulb through a fiber optic cable and is emitted from the sides and ends of the fibers inside a plastic pad. They work on the premise that phototherapy can be improved by delivering higher-intensity therapeutic light to decrease bilirubin levels. The pads do not produce appreciable heat like banks of lights or spotlights do, so insensible water loss is not increased. Eye patches also are not needed; thus, parents can feed and hold their newborns continuously to promote bonding.

4. The Moro reflex, or the embrace reflex, occurs when the neonate is startled. To elicit this reflex, the newborn is placed on his back. The upper body weight of the supine newborn is supported by the arms with use of a lifting motion, without lifting the newborn off the surface. When the arms are released suddenly, the newborn will throw the arms outward and flex the knees; arms then return to the chest. The fingers also spread to form a C. The newborn initially appears startled and then relaxes to a normal resting position.

5. Caput succedaneum is a localized edema on the scalp that occurs from the pressure of the birth process. It is commonly observed after prolonged labor. Clinically, it appears as a poorly demarcated soft tissue swelling that crosses suture lines. Pitting edema and overlying petechiae and ecchymosis are noted. The swelling will gradually dissipate in about 3 days without any treatment. Newborns who were

delivered via vacuum extraction usually have a caput in the area where the cup was used.

6. Erythema toxicum is a benign, idiopathic, very common, generalized, transient rash occurring in as many as 70% of all newborns during the first week of life. It consists of small papules or pustules on the skin resembling flea bites. The rash is common on the face, chest, and back. One of the chief characteristics of this rash is its lack of pattern. It is caused by the newborn's eosinophils reacting to the environment as the immune system matures. It does not require any treatment, and it disappears in a few days.

Activity F

1. a. The nurse should inform the mother that newborns usually sleep for up to 20 hours daily, for periods of 2 to 4 hours at a time, but not through the night. This is because their stomach capacity is too small to go long periods of time without nourishment. All newborns develop their own sleep patterns and cycles.

    b. The nurse should ask the mother to place the newborn on her back to sleep; remove all fluffy bedding, quilts, sheepskins, stuffed animals, and pillows from the crib to prevent potential suffocation. Parents should avoid unsafe conditions such as placing the newborn in the prone position, using a crib that does not meet federal safety guidelines, allowing window cords to hang loose and in close proximity to the crib, or having the room temperature too high, causing overheating.

    c. The nurse should educate Karen about potential risks of bed-sharing. Bringing a newborn into bed to nurse or quiet her down and then falling asleep with the newborn is not a safe practice. Infants who sleep in adult beds are up to 40 times more likely to suffocate than those who sleep in cribs. Suffocation also can occur when the infant gets entangled in bedding or caught under pillows, or slips between the bed and the wall or the headboard and mattress. It can also happen when someone accidentally rolls against or on top of them. Therefore, the safest sleeping location for all newborns is in their crib, without any movable objects close.

Activity G

1. **Answer: b**
    RATIONALE: The nurse should complete the second assessment for the newborn within the first 2 to 4 hours, when the newborn is in the nursery. The nurse should complete the initial newborn assessment in the birthing area and the third assessment before the newborn is discharged.

2. **Answer: d**
    RATIONALE: The nurse should place the newborn skin-to-skin with mother. This would help to maintain baby's temperature as well as promote breastfeeding and bonding between the mother and baby. The nurse can weigh the infant as long as a warmed cover is placed on the scale. The stethoscope should be warmed before it makes contact with the infant's skin, rather than using the stethoscope over the garment, because it may obscure the reading. The newborn's crib should not be placed close to the outer walls in the room to prevent heat loss through radiation.

3. **Answer: a**
    RATIONALE: Skin turgor is checked by pinching the skin over chest or abdomen and noting the return to original position; if the skin remains "tented" after pinching, it denotes dehydration. Stork bites or salmon patches, unopened sebaceous glands, and blue or purple splotches on buttocks are common skin variations not related to skin turgor.

4. **Answer: c**
    RATIONALE: As per the recommendations of AAP, all infants should receive a daily supplement of vitamin D during the first two months of life to prevent rickets and vitamin D deficiency. There is no need to feed the infant water, as breast milk contains enough water to meet the newborn's needs. Iron supplements need not be given, as the infant is being breastfed. Infants over six months of age are given fluoride supplementation if they are not receiving fluoridated water.

5. **Answer: a**
    RATIONALE: The nurse should instruct the woman to use the sealed and chilled milk within 24 hours. The nurse should not instruct the woman to use frozen milk within 6 months of obtaining it, to use microwave ovens to warm chilled milk, or to refreeze the used milk and reuse it. Instead, the nurse should instruct the woman to use frozen milk within 3 months of obtaining it, to avoid using microwave ovens to warm chilled milk, and to discard any used milk and never refreeze it.

6. **Answer: a**
    RATIONALE: The nurse should ask the mother to hold the baby upright with the baby's head on her mother's shoulder. Alternatively, the nurse can also suggest the mother sit with the newborn on her lap with the newborn lying face down. Gently rubbing the baby's abdomen or giving frequent sips of warm water to the infant will not significantly induce burping; burping is induced by the newborn's position.

7. **Answer: b**
    RATIONALE: The nurse should inform the client to introduce just one new single-ingredient food at a time to watch for allergies. The infant should not be coaxed to eat if he or she is not willing. Fruits should be introduced after cereals and before vegetables and eggs are introduced. A variety of solid foods should be introduced to provide a balanced diet.

8. **Answer: d**
    RATIONALE: A concentration of immature blood vessels causes salmon patches. Mongolian spots are caused by a concentration of pigmented cells and

usually disappear within the first 4 years of life. Erythema toxicum is caused by the newborn's eosinophils reacting to the environment as the immune system matures, and Harlequin sign is a result of immature autoregulation of blood flow and is commonly seen in low–birth-weight newborns.

9. **Answer: c**
RATIONALE: The nurse should obtain a newborn's temperature by placing an electronic temperature probe in the midaxillary area. The nurse should not tape an electronic thermistor probe to the abdominal skin, as this method is applied only when the newborn is placed under a radiant heat source. Rectal temperatures are no longer taken because of the risk of perforation. Oral temperature readings are not taken for newborns.

10. **Answer: c**
RATIONALE: The nurse should conclude that the newborn is facing moderate difficulty in adjusting to extrauterine life. The nurse need not conclude severe distress in adjusting to extrauterine life, better condition of the newborn, or abnormal central nervous system status. If the Apgar score is 8 points or higher, it indicates that the condition of the newborn is better. An Apgar score of 0 to 3 points represents severe distress in adjusting to extrauterine life.

11. **Answer: a**
RATIONALE: The nurse should instruct the parent to expose the newborn's bottom to air several times per day to prevent diaper rashes. Use of plastic pants and products such as powder and items with fragrance should be avoided. The parent should be instructed to place the newborn's buttocks in warm water after having had a diaper on all night.

12. **Answer: b, d, & e**
RATIONALE: The nurse should give the newborn oxygen, ensure the newborn's warmth, and observe the newborn's respiratory status frequently. The nurse need not give the infant warm water to drink or massage the infant's back.

13. **Answer: a, c, & e**
RATIONALE: The nurse should monitor the newborn for lethargy, cyanosis, and jitteriness. Low-pitched crying or rashes on the infant's skin are not signs generally associated with hypoglycemia.

14. **Answer: a, c, & e**
RATIONALE: To relieve breast engorgement in the client, the nurse should educate the client to take warm-to-hot showers to encourage milk release, express some milk manually before breastfeeding, and apply warm compresses to the breasts prior to nursing. The mother should be asked to feed the newborn in a variety of positions—sitting up and then lying down. The breasts should be massaged from under the axillary area, down toward the nipple.

15 **Answer: a, c, & e**
RATIONALE: Mongolian spots, swollen genitals in the female baby, and a short, creased neck are normal findings in a newborn. Mongolian spots are blue or

purple splotches that appear on the lower back and buttocks of newborns. Female babies may have swollen genitals as a result of maternal estrogen. The newborn's neck will appear almost nonexistent because it is so short. Creases are usually noted. Enlarged fontanelles are associated with malnutrition; hydrocephaly; congenital hypothyroidism; trisomies 13, 18, and 21; and various bone disorders such as osteogenesis imperfecta. Low-set ears are characteristic of many syndromes and genetic abnormalities such as trisomies 13 and 18 and internal organ abnormalities involving the renal system.

CHAPTER 19

Activity A

1. Oligohydramnios
2. Clonus
3. latent
4. hyperreflexia
5. incompatibility
6. Monozygotic
7. infection
8. spontaneous
9. first
10. Gestational

Activity B

1. **a.** Partial abruption with concealed hemorrhage.
   b. Partial abruption with apparent hemorrhage.
   c. Complete abruption with concealed hemorrhage.

Activity C

1. c   **2.** e   **3.** a   **4.** b   **5.** d

Activity D

1.

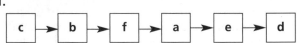

Activity E

1. Possible complications of hyperemesis gravidarum include persistent, uncontrollable nausea, dehydration, acid-base imbalances, electrolyte imbalances, and weight loss. If the condition is allowed to continue, it jeopardizes fetal well-being.
2. Conditions commonly associated with early bleeding (first half of pregnancy) include spontaneous abortion, ectopic pregnancy, and gestational trophoblastic disease (GTD).
3. Ectopic pregnancies usually result from conditions that obstruct or slow the passage of the fertilized ovum through the fallopian tube to the uterus. This may be a physical blockage in the tube or failure of the tubal epithelium to move the zygote (the cell formed after the egg is fertilized) down the tube into the uterus. In the general population, most cases are the result of tubal scarring

secondary to pelvic inflammatory disease. Organisms such as *Neisseria gonorrhoeae* and *Chlamydia trachomatis* preferentially attack the fallopian tubes, producing silent infections.

4. Risk factors for hyperemesis gravidarum include young age, nausea and vomiting with previous pregnancy, history of intolerance of oral contraceptives, nulliparity, trophoblastic disease, multiple gestation, emotional or psychological stress, gastroesophageal reflux disease, primigravida status, obesity, hyperthyroidism, and *Helicobacter pylori* seropositivity.

5. A nurse should include the following in prevention education for ectopic pregnancies:
   • Reducing risk factors such as sexual intercourse with multiple partners or intercourse without a condom
   • Avoiding contracting STIs that lead to pelvic inflammatory disease (PID)
   • Obtaining early diagnosis and adequate treatment of STIs
   • Avoiding the use of an IUC as a contraceptive method to reduce the risk of repeat ascending infections responsible for tubal scarring
   • Using condoms to decrease the risk of infections that cause tubal scarring
   • Seeking prenatal care early if pregnant, to confirm location of pregnancy

6. The Kleihauer–Betke test detects fetal RBCs in the maternal circulation, determines the degree of fetal–maternal hemorrhage, and helps calculate the appropriate dosage of RhoGAM to give for Rh-negative clients.

Activity F

1. **a.** Recognizing preterm labor at an early stage requires that the expectant mother and her health care team identify the subtle symptoms of preterm labor. These may include
   • Change or increase in vaginal discharge
   • Pelvic pressure (pushing down sensation)
   • Low, dull backache
   • Menstrual-like cramps
   • Uterine contractions, with or without pain
   • Intestinal cramping, with or without diarrhea
   b. The nurse must teach Jenna how to palpate and time uterine contractions. Provide written materials to support this education at a level and in a language appropriate for her. Also, educate Jenna about the importance of prenatal care, risk reduction, and recognizing the signs and symptoms of preterm labor. The nurse may also include
   • Stressing good hydration and consumption of a nutritious diet
   • Advising against any activity, such as sexual activity or nipple stimulation, that might stimulate oxytocin release and initiate uterine contractions
   • Assessing stress levels of client and family, and making appropriate referrals

   • Providing emotional support and client empowerment throughout
   • Emphasizing the possible need for more frequent office visits and for notifying the health care provider if she has questions or concerns.

Activity G

1. **Answer: c**
   RATIONALE: The nurse should instruct the client with hyperemesis gravidarum to eat small, frequent meals throughout the day to minimize nausea and vomiting. The nurse should also instruct the client to avoid lying down or reclining for at least two hours after eating and to increase the intake of carbonated beverages. The nurse should instruct the client to try foods that settle the stomach such as dry crackers, toast, or soda.

2. **Answer: a**
   RATIONALE: A temperature elevation or an increase in the pulse of a client with PROM would indicate infection. Increase in the pulse does not indicate preterm labor or cord compression. The nurse should monitor fetal heart rate patterns continuously, reporting any variable decelerations suggesting cord compression. Respiratory distress syndrome is one of the perinatal risks associated with PROM.

3. **Answer: c**
   RATIONALE: The nurse should closely assess the woman for hemorrhage after giving birth by frequently assessing uterine involution. Assessing skin turgor and blood pressure and monitoring hCG titers will not help to determine hemorrhage.

4. **Answer: b**
   RATIONALE: When meconium is present in the amniotic fluid, it typically indicates fetal distress related to hypoxia. Meconium stains the fluid yellow to greenish brown, depending on the amount present. A decreased amount of amniotic fluid reduces the cushioning effect, thereby making cord compression a possibility. A foul odor of amniotic fluid indicates infection. Meconium in the amniotic fluid does not indicate CNS involvement.

5. **Answer: d**
   RATIONALE: The nurse should institute and maintain seizure precautions such as padding the side rails and having oxygen, suction equipment, and call light readily available to protect the client from injury. The nurse should provide a quiet, darkened room to stabilize the client. The nurse should maintain the client on complete bed rest in the left lateral lying position and not in a supine position. Keeping the head of the bed slightly elevated will not help maintain seizure precautions.

6. **Answer: a**
   RATIONALE: If the client is receiving magnesium sulfate to suppress or control seizures, assess deep tendon reflexes to determine the effectiveness of therapy. Common sites utilized to assess DTRs are the biceps reflex, triceps reflex, patellar reflex,

Achilles reflex, and plantar reflex. Assessing the mucous membranes for dryness and skin turgor for dehydration are the required interventions when caring for a client with hyperemesis gravidarum. Monitoring intake and output will not help to determine the effectiveness of therapy.

7. **Answer: d**

RATIONALE: A previous myomectomy to remove fibroids can be associated with the cause of placenta previa. Risk factors also include advanced maternal age (greater than 30 years old). A structurally defective cervix cannot be associated with the cause of placenta previa. However, it can be associated with the cause of cervical insufficiency. Alcohol ingestion is not a risk factor for developing placenta previa but is associated with abruptio placenta.

8. **Answer: b**

RATIONALE: The nurse should encourage a client with mild elevations in blood pressure to rest as much as possible in the lateral recumbent position to improve uteroplacental blood flow, reduce blood pressure, and promote diuresis. The nurse should maintain the client with severe preeclampsia on complete bed rest in the left lateral lying position. Keeping the head of the bed slightly elevated will not help to improve the condition of the client with mild elevations in blood pressure.

9. **Answer: d**

RATIONALE: The first choice for fluid replacement is generally 5% dextrose in lactated Ringer's solution with vitamins and electrolytes added. If the client does not improve after several days of bed rest, "gut rest," IV fluids, and antiemetics, then total parenteral nutrition (TPN) or percutaneous endoscopic gastrostomy (PEG) tube feeding is instituted to prevent malnutrition.

10. **Answer: c**

RATIONALE: The classic manifestations of abruptio placenta are painful dark red vaginal bleeding, "knife-like" abdominal pain, uterine tenderness, contractions, and decreased fetal movement. Painless bright red vaginal bleeding is the clinical manifestation of placenta previa. Generalized vasospasm is the clinical manifestation of preeclampsia and not of abruptio placenta.

11. **Answer: a**

RATIONALE: The symptoms if rupture or hemorrhaging occurs before successfully treating the pregnancy are lower abdomen pain, feelings of faintness, phrenic nerve irritation, hypotension, marked abdominal tenderness with distension, and hypovolemic shock. Painless bright red vaginal bleeding occurring during the second or third trimester is the clinical manifestation of placenta previa. Fetal distress and tetanic contractions are not the symptoms observed in a client if rupture or hemorrhaging occurs before successfully treating an ectopic pregnancy.

12. **Answer: d**

RATIONALE: When the woman arrives and is admitted, assessing her vital signs, the amount and color of the bleeding, and current pain rating on a scale of 1 to 10 are the priorities. Assessing the signs of shock, monitoring uterine contractility, and determining the amount of funneling are not priority assessments when a pregnant woman complaining of vaginal bleeding is admitted to the hospital.

13. **Answer: c**

RATIONALE: A nurse should closely monitor the client's vital signs, bleeding (peritoneal or vaginal) to identify hypovolemic shock that may occur with tubal rupture. Beta-hCG level is monitored to diagnose an ectopic pregnancy or impending abortion. Monitoring the mass with transvaginal ultrasound (TVS) and determining the size of the mass are done for diagnosing an ectopic pregnancy. Monitoring the fetal heart rate does not help to identify hypovolemic shock.

14. **Answer: a**

RATIONALE: The current recommendation is that every Rh-negative nonimmunized woman receives Rho-GAM at 28 weeks' gestation and again within 72 hours after giving birth. Consuming a well-balanced nutritional diet and avoiding sexual activity until after 28 weeks will not help to prevent complications of blood incompatibility. Transvaginal ultrasound helps to validate the position of the placenta and will not help to prevent complications of blood incompatibility.

15. **Answer: c**

RATIONALE: The nurse should know that coma usually follows an eclamptic seizure. Muscle rigidity occurs after facial twitching. Respirations do not become rapid during the seizure; they cease. Coma usually follows the seizure activity, with respiration resuming.

16. **Answer: d**

RATIONALE: The nurse should know that dependent edema may be seen in the sacral area if the client is on bed rest. Pitting edema leaves a small depression or pit after finger pressure is applied to a swollen area and can be measured. This is not possible in dependent edema. Dependent edema may occur in clients who are both ambulatory and on bed rest.

17. **Answer: a, c, & d**

RATIONALE: Signs such as a change or increase in vaginal discharge, rupture of membranes, and uterine contractions should be further assessed as a possible sign of preterm labor. Phrenic nerve irritation and hypovolemic shock are the symptoms if rupture or hemorrhaging occurs before successfully treating the ectopic pregnancy.

18. **Answer: a, b, & e**

RATIONALE: The associated conditions and complications of premature rupture of the membranes are infection, prolapsed cord, abruptio placenta, and preterm labor. Spontaneous abortion and placenta previa are not associated conditions or complications of premature rupture of the membranes.

19. **Answer: b, d, & e**
    RATIONALE: The signs and symptoms of HELLP syndrome are nausea, malaise, epigastric pain, upper right quadrant pain, demonstrable edema, and hyperbilirubinemia. Blood pressure higher than 160/110 and oliguria are the symptoms of severe preeclampsia rather than HELLP syndrome.

20. **Answer: b, d, & e**
    RATIONALE: Adverse effects commonly associated with misoprostol include dyspepsia, hypotension, tachycardia, diarrhea, abdominal pain, and vomiting. Constipation and headache are not adverse effects commonly associated with misoprostol.

CHAPTER 20

Activity A

1. somatotropin
2. Gestational
3. airway
4. lung
5. Anemia
6. bacterium
7. Toxoplasmosis
8. Adolescence
9. Nicotine
10. Cocaine

Activity B

1. **a.** This disorder is known as fetal alcohol spectrum disorder, which includes a full range of birth defects, such as structural anomalies and behavioral and neurocognitive disabilities caused by prenatal exposure to alcohol.

   b. Characteristics of fetal alcohol spectrum disorder include craniofacial dysmorphia (thin upper lip, small head circumference, and small eyes), intrauterine growth restriction, microcephaly, and congenital anomalies such as limb abnormalities and cardiac defects.

Activity C

1. f   2. e   3. d   4. c   5. b
6. a

Activity D

1. The most common complications in a pregnant client with hypertension are
   - Increased risk for developing preeclampsia
   - Fetal growth restriction during pregnancy
2. The nurse should include the following elements during the physical examination of pregnant clients with asthma:
   - Rate, rhythm, and depth of respirations
   - Skin color
   - Blood pressure
   - Pulse rate
   - Evaluation for signs of fatigue

3. The nurse should include the following factors in the teaching plan for a client with asthma:
   - Signs and symptoms of asthma progression and exacerbation
   - Importance and safety of medication to fetus and to herself
   - Warning signs; potential harm to fetus and self by undertreatment or delay in seeking help
   - Prevention and avoidance of known triggers
   - Home use of metered-dose inhalers
   - Adverse effects of medications

4. Assessment of tuberculosis in pregnant clients includes the following:
   - At antepartum visits, the nurse should be alert for clinical manifestations of tuberculosis such as fatigue, fever or night sweats, nonproductive cough, slow weight loss, anemia, hemoptysis, and anorexia
   - If tuberculosis is suspected or the woman is at risk for developing tuberculosis, the nurse should anticipate screening with purified protein derivative (PPD) administered by intradermal injection; if the client has been exposed to tuberculosis, a reddened induration will appear within 72 hours
   - A follow-up chest x-ray with a lead shield over the abdomen and sputum cultures will confirm the diagnosis

5. The developmental tasks associated with adolescent behavior are
   - Seeking economic and social stability
   - Developing a personal value system
   - Building meaningful relationships with others
   - Becoming comfortable with their changing bodies
   - Working to become independent from their parents
   - Learning to verbalize conceptually

6. The effects of sedatives by the mother on her infant are as follows:
   - Sedatives easily cross the placenta and cause birth defects and behavioral problems
   - Infants born to mothers who abuse sedatives may be physically dependent on the drugs and prone to respiratory problems, feeding difficulties, disturbed sleep, sweating, irritability, and fever

Activity E

1. **a.** The greatest increase in asthma attacks in the pregnant client usually occurs between 24 and 36 weeks' gestation; flare-ups are rare during the last four weeks of pregnancy and during labor.

   b. Successful management of asthma in pregnancy involves
   - Drug therapy
   - Client education
   - Elimination of environmental triggers

   c. The following are the nursing interventions involved when caring for the pregnant client with asthma during labor:
   - Monitor client's oxygen saturation by pulse oximetry

- Provide pain management through epidural analgesia
- Continuously monitor the fetus for distress during labor and assess fetal heart rate patterns for indications of hypoxia
- Assess the newborn for signs and symptoms of hypoxia

Activity F

1. Answer: b

RATIONALE: The nurse should identify postprandial hyperglycemia as the effect of insulin resistance in the client. Hypertension, hypercholesterolemia, and myocardial infarction are not the effects of insulin resistance in a diabetic client.

2. Answer: a

RATIONALE: The nurse should identify respiratory distress syndrome as a major risk that can be faced by the offspring of a client with cardiovascular disease. Congenital varicella syndrome can occur in an offspring of a mother infected with varicella during early pregnancy. Sudden infant death syndrome can occur in an offspring of a mother who smokes during pregnancy. Prune belly syndrome is a fetal anomaly associated with cocaine use in early pregnancy.

3. Answer: b

RATIONALE: The nurse should stress the positive benefits of a healthy lifestyle during the preconception counseling of a client with chronic hypertension. The client need not avoid dairy products or increase intake of vitamin D supplements. It may not be advisable for a client with chronic hypertension to exercise without consultation.

4. Answer: a

RATIONALE: Swelling of the face is a symptom of cardiac decompensation, along with moist, frequent cough and rapid respirations. Dry, rasping cough; slow, labored respiration; and an elevated temperature are not symptoms of cardiac decompensation.

5. Answer: d

RATIONALE: The nurse should assess the client with heart disease for cardiac decompensation, which is most common from 28 to 32 weeks of gestation and in the first 48 hours postpartum. Limiting sodium intake, inspecting the extremities for edema, and ensuring that the client consumes a high-fiber diet are interventions during pregnancy, not in the first 48 hours postpartum.

6. Answer: b

RATIONALE: The nurse should evaluate for signs of fatigue during the physical examination of a client with asthma. The nurse need not monitor the client's temperature, frequency of headache, or feelings of nausea, because these conditions are not related to asthma.

7. Answer: a

RATIONALE: The nurse should instruct the pregnant client with tuberculosis to maintain adequate hydration as a health-promoting activity. The

client need not avoid direct sunlight or red meat, or wear light clothes; these have no impact on the client's condition.

8. Answer: c

RATIONALE: The nurse should identify preterm birth as a risk associated with anemia during pregnancy. Anemia during pregnancy does not increase the risk of a newborn with heart problems, an enlarged liver, or fetal asphyxia.

9. Answer: b

RATIONALE: The nurse should assess for possible fluid overload in a client with cardiovascular disease who has just delivered. The nurse need not assess for shortness of breath or edema or auscultate heart sounds for abnormalities. It is important for the nurse to assess for edema and note any pitting and auscultate heart sounds for abnormalities during the antepartum period to ensure early detection of cardiac decompensation.

10. Answer: a

RATIONALE: The nurse should stress the importance of good handwashing and use of sound hygiene practices to reduce transmission of the virus to a client who could pass the virus on to her fetus. Drinking plenty of fluids will not help minimize this risk. The client need not take antibiotics if she has not been infected. It is not practical for the client to avoid interaction with children.

11. Answer: d

RATIONALE: The nurse should address the client's knowledge of child development during assessment of the pregnant adolescent client. The nurse need not address the sexual development of the client, whether sex was consensual, or the stress levels of the client.

12. Answer: a

RATIONALE: The nurse should inform the client that she could be at risk for coronary artery disease because medical conditions such as coronary artery disease and myocardial infarction may result in the older pregnant woman. The nurse need not ask the client to avoid excessive exposure to sunlight or consumption of poultry. The nurse should not ask the client to perform aerobic exercises if the client is not accustomed to exercising.

13. Answer: d

RATIONALE: The nurse should stress the avoidance of breastfeeding when counseling a pregnant client who is HIV-positive. The nurse need not discuss the client's relationship with the spouse. The client can be taught gradually about care to be taken during physical contact with the infant or when visiting crowded places.

14. Answer: b

RATIONALE: The nurse should caution the client about high levels of anxiety as a risk associated with substance abuse during pregnancy. Substance abuse does not increase the risk of post-term birth, stillbirth, or transient tachypnea of the newborn.

15. Answer: b
RATIONALE: The nurse should make the client aware of increased risk of anemia as a possible effect of maternal coffee consumption during pregnancy, as it decreases iron absorption. Maternal coffee consumption during pregnancy does not increase the risk of heart disease, rickets, or scurvy.

16. Answer: a, b, & e
RATIONALE: To minimize risk of toxoplasmosis, the nurse should instruct the client to eat meat that has been cooked to an internal temperature of 160°F throughout and to avoid cleaning the cat's litter box or performing activities such as gardening. The client should avoid feeding the cat raw or undercooked meat. The cat should be kept indoors to prevent it from hunting and eating birds or rodents.

17. Answer: c, d, & e
RATIONALE: Obesity, hypertension, and a previous infant weighing more than 9 pounds are risk factors for developing gestational diabetes. Maternal age less than 18 years and genitourinary tract abnormalities do not increase the risk of developing gestational diabetes.

18. Answer: a, d, & e
RATIONALE: The nurse caring for a pregnant client with sickle cell anemia should teach the client meticulous handwashing to prevent the risk of infection, assess the hydration status of the client at each visit, and urge the client to drink 8 to 10 glasses of fluid daily. The nurse need not assess serum electrolyte levels of the client at each visit or instruct the client to consume protein-rich food.

19. Answer: a
RATIONALE: The nurse should assess for small head circumference in a newborn being assessed for fetal alcohol spectrum disorder. Fetal alcohol spectrum disorder does not cause decreased blood glucose level, a poor breathing pattern, or wide eyes.

20. Answer: b
RATIONALE: The nurse should stress the inclusion of complex carbohydrates in the diet in the dietary plan for a pregnant woman with pregestational diabetes. The pregnant client with pregestational diabetes need not include more dairy products in the diet, eat only two meals per day, or eat at least one egg per day; these have no impact on the client's condition.

CHAPTER 21

Activity A
1. dystocia
2. Breech
3. Leopold's
4. Tocolytic
5. Steroids
6. fibronectin
7. Bishop
8. Hygroscopic
9. amniotomy
10. Oxytocin

Activity B
1. The figures depict various maneuvers to relieve shoulder dystocia. A. McRobert's maneuver. The mother's thighs are flexed and abducted as much as possible to straighten the pelvic curve. B. Suprapubic pressure. Pressure is applied just above the pubic bone, pushing the fetal anterior shoulder downward to displace it from above the mother's symphysis pubis. The newborn's head is depressed toward the maternal anus while suprapubic pressure is applied.
2. The figures depict prolapsed cord. A. Prolapse within the uterus. B. Prolapse with the cord visible at the vulva.

Activity C
1. c   **2.** a   **3.** e   **4.** b   **5.** d

Activity D
1.

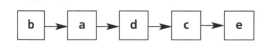

Activity E
1. The symptoms of preterm labor are
   - Change or increase in vaginal discharge
   - Pelvic pressure (pushing down sensation)
   - Low, dull backache
   - Menstrual-like cramps
   - Heaviness or aching in the thighs
   - Uterine contractions, with or without pain
   - Intestinal cramping, with or without diarrhea
2. Cervical ripeness is an assessment of the readiness of the cervix to efface and dilate in response to uterine contractions. It is an important variable when labor induction is being considered. A ripe cervix is shortened, centered (anterior), softened, and partially dilated. An unripe cervix is long, closed, posterior, and firm. Cervical ripening usually begins prior to the onset of labor contractions and is necessary for cervical dilatation and the passage of the fetus.
3. Uterine rupture is a catastrophic tearing of the uterus at the site of a previous scar into the abdominal cavity. The onset is often marked only by sudden fetal bradycardia, and the obliteration of intrauterine pressure/cessation of contractions. Treatment requires rapid surgical attention. In uterine rupture, fetal morbidity occurs secondary to catastrophic hemorrhage, fetal anoxia, or both.
4. Indications of amnioinfusion are severe variable decelerations due to cord compression, oligohydramnios due to placental insufficiency, postmaturity or rupture of membranes, preterm labor with premature rupture of membranes, and thick meconium

fluid. Vaginal bleeding of unknown origin, umbilical cord prolapse, amnionitis, uterine hypertonicity, and severe fetal distress are contraindications to amnioinfusion.

5. The nurse assesses each client to help predict her risk status. The nurse should be aware that cord prolapse is more common in pregnancies involving malpresentation, growth restriction, prematurity, ruptured membranes with a fetus at a high station, hydramnios, grand multiparity, and multifetal gestation. The client and fetus should be thoroughly assessed to detect changes and evaluate the effectiveness of any interventions performed.

6. Shoulder dystocia can cause postpartum hemorrhage, secondary to uterine atony or vaginal lacerations in the mother. In the fetus, shoulder dystocia can result in transient and/or permanent Erb or Duchenne brachial plexus palsies and clavicular or humeral fractures, as well as hypoxic encephalopathy.

Activity F

1. The nurse should perform the following interventions during amnioinfusion to prevent maternal and fetal complications:
   - Explain the need for the procedure, what it involves, and how it may solve the problem
   - Inform the mother that she will need to remain on bed rest during the procedure
   - Assess the mother's vital signs and associated discomfort level
   - Maintain adequate intake and output records
   - Assess the duration and intensity of uterine contractions frequently to identify overdistention or increased uterine tone
   - Monitor FHR pattern to determine whether the amnioinfusion is improving the fetal status
   - Prepare the mother for a possible cesarean birth if the FHR does not improve after the amnioinfusion

Activity G

1. **Answer: a**
   RATIONALE: A forceps and vacuum–assisted birth is required for the client having a prolonged second stage of labor. In cases of uterine rupture, the baby has to be immediately delivered by cesarean section. Oligohydramnios due to placental insufficiency and preterm labor with premature rupture of membranes are treated with amnioinfusion.

2. **Answer: d**
   RATIONALE: The nurse should know that gestational hypertension leads to placental abruption. Other factors leading to placental abruption include preeclampsia, seizure activity, uterine rupture, trauma, smoking, cocaine use, coagulation defects, previous history of abruption, domestic violence, and placental pathology. These conditions may force blood into the under layer of the placenta and cause it to detach. Gestational diabetes, cardiovascular disease, and excess weight gain during

pregnancy, though dangerous conditions, are not known to specifically cause placental abruption.

3. **Answer: a**
   RATIONALE: The nurse should monitor cyanosis when caring for a client with amniotic fluid embolism. Other signs and symptoms of this condition include hypotension, cyanosis, seizures, tachycardia, coagulation failure, disseminated intravascular coagulation, pulmonary edema, uterine atony with subsequent hemorrhage, adult respiratory distress syndrome, and cardiac arrest. Arrhythmia, hematuria, and hyperglycemia are not known to occur in cases of amniotic fluid embolism. Hematuria is seen in clients having uterine rupture.

4. **Answer: a**
   RATIONALE: Chorioamnionitis is an indication for labor induction. Complete placenta previa, abruptio placenta, and transverse fetal lie are contraindications for labor induction.

5. **Answer: a**
   RATIONALE: The nurse should ensure that the client does not have uterine hypertonicity to confirm that amnioinfusion is not contraindicated. Other factors that enforce contraindication of amnioinfusion include vaginal bleeding of unknown origin, umbilical cord prolapse, amnionitis, and severe fetal distress. Active genital herpes infection, abruptio placentae, and invasive cervical cancer are conditions that enforce contraindication of labor induction rather than amnioinfusion.

6. **Answer: d**
   RATIONALE: The nurse should identify nerve damage as a risk to the fetus in cases of shoulder dystocia. Other fetal risks include asphyxia, clavicle fracture, central nervous system (CNS) injury or dysfunction, and death. Bladder injury, infection, and extensive lacerations are poor maternal outcomes due to the occurrence of shoulder dystocia.

7. **Answer: a**
   RATIONALE: A Bishop score of less than six indicates that a cervical ripening method should be used before inducing labor. A low Bishop score is not an indication for cesarean birth; there are several other factors that need to be considered for a cesarean birth. A Bishop score of less than six indicates that vaginal birth will be unsuccessful and prolonged, because the duration of labor is inversely correlated with the Bishop score.

8. **Answer: a**
   RATIONALE: When caring for a client who has undergone a cesarean section, the nurse should assess the client's uterine tone to determine fundal firmness. The nurse should assist with breastfeeding initiation and offer continued support. The nurse can also suggest alternate positioning techniques to reduce incisional discomfort while breastfeeding. Delaying breastfeeding may not be required. The nurse should encourage the

client to cough, perform deep-breathing exercises, and use the incentive spirometer every 2 hours. The nurse should assist the client with early ambulation to prevent respiratory and cardiovascular problems.

9. **Answer: d**
RATIONALE: Overdistended uterus is a contraindication for oxytocin administration. Post-term status, dysfunctional labor pattern, and prolonged ruptured membranes are indications for administration of oxytocin.

10. **Answer: a**
RATIONALE: The nurse caring for the client in labor with shoulder dystocia of the fetus should assist with positioning the client in squatting position. The client can also be helped into the hands and knees position or lateral recumbent position for birth, to free the shoulders. Assessing for complaints of intense back pain in first stage of labor, anticipating possible use of forceps to rotate to anterior position at birth, and assessing for prolonged second stage of labor with arrest of descent are important interventions when caring for a client with persistent occiput posterior position of fetus.

11. **Answer: a**
RATIONALE: The nurse should assess infertility treatment as a contributor to increased probability of multiple gestations. Multiple gestations do not occur with an adolescent delivery; instead, chances of multiple gestations are known to increase due to the increasing number of women giving birth at older ages. Medications and advanced maternal age are not known to cause multiple gestations.

12. **Answer: d**
RATIONALE: Cephalopelvic disproportion is associated with post-term pregnancy. Underdeveloped suck reflex, congenital heart defects, and intraventricular hemorrhage are associated with preterm pregnancy.

13. **Answer: c**
RATIONALE: The nurse should assess for fetal complications such as head trauma associated with intracranial hemorrhage, nerve damage, and hypoxia in cases of precipitous labor. Facial and scalp lacerations, facial nerve injury, and cephalhematoma are all newborn traumas associated with the use of the forceps of vacuum extractors during birth. These conditions are not neonatal complications associated with precipitous labor.

14. **Answer: c**
RATIONALE: Prolonged pregnancy is the cause of intrauterine fetal demise in late pregnancy that the nurse should be aware of. Other factors resulting in intrauterine fetal demise include infection, hypertension, advanced maternal age, Rh disease, uterine rupture, diabetes, congenital anomalies, cord accident, abruption, premature rupture of membranes, or hemorrhage. Hydramnios, multifetal gestation, and malpresentation are not the

causes of intrauterine fetal demise in late pregnancy; they are causes of umbilical cord prolapse.

15. **Answer: a**
RATIONALE: The nurse should monitor for fetal hypoxia in cases of umbilical cord prolapse. Because this is the fetus's only lifeline, fetal perfusion deteriorates rapidly. Complete occlusion renders the fetus helpless and oxygen-deprived. Preeclampsia, coagulation defects, and placental pathology are not risks associated with umbilical cord prolapse.

CHAPTER 22

Activity A
1. atony
2. Subinvolution
3. decrease
4. thrombus
5. thromboembolism
6. Metritis
7. mastitis
8. early
9. accreta
10. inversion

Activity B
1. The figure shows perineal hematoma with a bulging swollen mass.
2. The figure depicts postpartum wound infections: A, infected episiotomy site; B, infected cesarean birth incision.

Activity C
1. b   2. a   3. d   4. c

Activity D
1. Overdistention of the uterus can be caused by multifetal gestation, fetal macrosomia, polyhydramnios, fetal abnormality, or placental fragments. Other causes might include prolonged or rapid, forceful labor, especially if stimulated; bacterial toxins; use of anesthesia; and magnesium sulfate used in the treatment of preeclampsia. Overdistention of the uterus is a major risk factor for uterine atony, the most common cause of early postpartum hemorrhage, which can lead to hypovolemic shock.
2. Idiopathic thrombocytopenia purpura (ITP) is characterized by increased platelet destruction caused by the development of autoantibodies to platelet-membrane antigens. The incidence of ITP in adults is approximately 66 cases per 1 million per year. The characteristic features of the disorder are thrombocytopenia, capillary fragility, and increased bleeding time. Clients with ITP present with easy bruising, bleeding from mucous membranes, menorrhagia, epistaxis, bleeding gums, hematomas, and severe hemorrhage after a cesarean birth or lacerations.
3. Postpartum infections are usually polymicrobial and involve *Staphylococcus aureus*, *Escherichia coli*,

Klebsiella species, *Gardnerella vaginalis,* gonococci, coliform bacteria, group A or B hemolytic streptococci, *Chlamydia trachomatis,* and the anaerobes that are common to bacterial vaginosis.

4. Most postpartum women experience baby blues. The woman exhibits mild depressive symptoms of anxiety, irritability, mood swings, tearfulness, and increased sensitivity, feelings of being overwhelmed, and fatigue after the birth of the baby. The condition typically peaks on postpartum days 4 and 5 and usually resolves by postpartum day 10. Baby blues are usually self-limiting and require no formal treatment other than reassurance and validation of the woman's experience, as well as assistance in caring for herself and the newborn.

5. Symptoms of postpartum psychosis surface within three weeks of giving birth. The main symptoms include sleep disturbances, fatigue, depression, and hypomania. The mother will be tearful, confused, and preoccupied with feelings of guilt and worthlessness. The symptoms may escalate to delirium, hallucinations, anger toward herself and her infant, bizarre behavior, manifestations of mania, and thoughts of hurting herself and the infant. The mother frequently loses touch with reality and experiences a severe regressive breakdown, associated with a high risk of suicide or infanticide.

6. A thrombosis refers to the development of a blood clot in the blood vessel. It can cause an inflammation of the blood vessel lining, which in turn can lead to a possible thromboembolism. Thrombi can involve the superficial or deep veins in the legs or pelvis:
   - Superficial venous thrombosis usually involves the saphenous venous system and is confined to the lower leg. The lithotomy position during birth can cause superficial thrombophlebitis in some women.
   - Deep venous thrombosis can involve deep veins from the foot to the calf, to the thighs, or to the pelvis.
   In both locations, thrombi can dislodge and migrate to the lungs, causing a pulmonary embolism.

Activity E

1. a. The major causes of thrombus formation are venous stasis, injury to the innermost layer of the blood vessel, and hypercoagulation. Venous stasis and hypercoagulation are common in the postpartum period. The risk factors for thrombosis are
   - Prolonged bed rest
   - Diabetes
   - Obesity
   - Cesarean birth
   - Smoking
   - Severe anemia
   - History of previous thrombosis
   - Varicose veins

   - Advanced maternal age (greater than 35 years)
   - Multiparity
   - Use of oral contraceptives before pregnancy

   b. The nurse should perform the following nursing interventions to prevent thromboembolic complications in a client:
   - Educate the client on the need for early and frequent ambulation
   - Encourage activities that cause leg muscles to contract (leg exercises and walking) to promote venous return in order to prevent venous stasis
   - Use intermittent sequential compression devices, which cause passive leg contractions. until the client is ambulatory
   - Elevate the client's leg above heart level to promote venous return
   - Ensure stockings are applied and removed every day for inspections of the legs
   - Encourage the client to perform passive exercises on the bed
   - Ensure that the client is involved in postoperative deep-breathing exercises; this improves venous return
   - In order to prevent venous pooling, avoid placing pillows under the knees or keeping the legs in stirrups for a long time
   - Ensure the use of bed cradles; this helps in keeping linens and blankets off the extremity

   c. For clients with superficial venous thrombosis, the nurse should perform the following interventions:
   - Administer NSAIDs for analgesic effect
   - Provide rest and elevation of the affected leg
   - Apply warm compresses over the affected area to promote healing
   - Use anti-embolism stockings, which promote circulation to the extremities

Activity F

1. **Answer: c**
   RATIONALE: The nurse should monitor the client for swelling in the calf. Swelling in the calf, erythema, and pedal edema are early manifestations of deep venous thrombosis, which may lead to pulmonary embolism if not prevented at an early stage. Sudden change in the mental status, difficulty in breathing, and sudden chest pain are manifestations of pulmonary embolism, beyond the stage of prevention.

2. **Answer: d**
   RATIONALE: When caring for a client with deep vein thrombosis (DVT), the nurse should instruct the client to avoid using oral contraceptives. Cigarette smoking, use of oral contraceptives, a sedentary lifestyle, and obesity increase the risk for developing DVT. The nurse should encourage the client with deep vein thrombosis to wear compression stockings. The nurse should instruct the client to avoid using products containing aspirin when

caring for clients with bleeding, but not for clients with DVT. Prolonged bed rest should be avoided. Prolonged bed rest involves staying motionless; this could lead to venous stasis, which needs to be avoided in cases of DVT.

3. **Answer: b**
RATIONALE: When caring for a client with idiopathic thrombocytopenic purpura, the nurse should administer platelet transfusions as ordered to control bleeding. Glucocorticoids, intravenous immunoglobulins, and intravenous anti-Rho D are also administered to the client. The nurse should not administer NSAIDs when caring for this client since nonsteroidal anti-inflammatory drugs cause platelet dysfunction. ITP is a disorder of increased platelet destruction due to the presence of autoantibodies to platelet-membrane antigens. As the client is bleeding, the nurse should continue with the administration of oxytocics, which helps to control the bleeding. Continuous firm uterine massage results in uterine exhaustion, leading to augmentation of bleeding.

4. **Answer: a**
RATIONALE: The nurse should monitor for foul-smelling vaginal discharge to verify the presence of an episiotomy infection. Sudden onset of shortness of breath, sudden change in mental status, and apprehension and diaphoresis are signs of pulmonary embolism and do not indicate episiotomy infection.

5. **Answer: a**
RATIONALE: The nurse should assess the client for prolonged bleeding time. von Willebrand disease (vWD) is a congenital bleeding disorder, inherited as an autosomal dominant trait, that is characterized by a prolonged bleeding time, a deficiency of von Willebrand factor, and impairment of platelet adhesion. A fever of 100.4°F after the first 24 hours after childbirth and presence of foul-smelling vaginal discharge indicate infection. A client with a postpartum fundal height that is higher than expected may have subinvolution of the uterus.

6. **Answer: d**
RATIONALE: The nurse should assess for calf tenderness in the client to verify the diagnosis of a deep vein thrombosis. Other signs and symptoms of deep vein thrombosis include calf swelling, erythema, warmth and tenderness, and pedal edema. Sudden chest pain, dyspnea, and tachypnea are signs and symptoms associated with pulmonary embolism and not deep vein thrombosis.

7. **Answer: d**
RATIONALE: The presence of a large uterus with painless dark-red blood mixed with clots indicates retained placental fragments in the uterus. This cause of hemorrhage can be prevented by carefully inspecting the placenta for intactness. A firm uterus with a trickle or steady stream of bright-red blood in the perineum indicates bleeding from trauma. A soft and boggy uterus that deviates from

the midline indicates a full bladder, interfering with uterine involution.

8. **Answer: a**
RATIONALE: The nurse can identify if the bleeding is from lacerations by looking for a well-contracted uterus with bright-red vaginal bleeding. Lacerations commonly occur during forceps delivery. In subinvolution of the uterus, there is inadequate contraction, resulting in bleeding. A boggy uterus with vaginal bleeding is seen in uterine atony. An inverted uterus with vaginal bleeding is seen in uterine inversion.

9. **Answer: c**
RATIONALE: Early postpartal hemorrhage can be assessed within the first few hours following delivery. Postpartal infection may be noticed as a rise in temperature after the first 24 hours following childbirth. Postpartal blues and postpartum depression are emotional disorders noticed much later, in the weeks following delivery.

10. **Answer: c**
RATIONALE: To help prevent the occurrence of postpartum thromboembolic complications, the nurse should instruct the client to avoid sitting or standing in one position for long periods of time. This prevents venous pooling. The nurse should instruct the client to perform postoperative deep-breathing exercises to improve venous return by relieving the negative thoracic pressure on leg veins. The nurse should instruct the client to prevent venous pooling by avoiding the use of pillows under the knees. Elevating the legs above heart level promotes venous return, and therefore the nurse should encourage it.

11. **Answer: c**
RATIONALE: A nurse should monitor for decreased blood pressure when evaluating the client for signs of hemorrhage. A falling blood pressure along with increased heart rate and decreased urinary output are the typical signs of severe hemorrhage. The client will also experience reduced, not increased, body temperature during hemorrhage.

12. **Answer: b**
RATIONALE: The nurse should educate the client to perform hand-washing before and after breastfeeding to prevent mastitis. Discontinuing breastfeeding to allow time for healing, avoiding hot or cold compresses on the breast, and discouraging manual compression of breast for expressing milk are inappropriate interventions. The nurse should educate the client to continue breastfeeding, because it reverses milk stasis, and to manually compress the breast to express excess milk. Hot and cold compresses can be applied for comfort.

13. **Answer: b, c, & d**
RATIONALE: The nurse should monitor for bleeding gums, tachycardia, and acute renal failure to assess for an increased risk of disseminated intravascular coagulation in the client. The other clinical manifestations of this condition include petechiae,

ecchymosis, and uncontrolled bleeding during birth. Hypotension and amount of lochia greater than usual are findings that might suggest a coagulopathy.

14. **Answer: a, b, & d**
    RATIONALE: The nurse should monitor the client for symptoms such as inability to concentrate, loss of confidence, and decreased interest in life to verify the presence of postpartum depression. Manifestations of mania and bizarre behavior are noted in clients with postpartum psychosis.

15. **Answer: a, b, & d**
    RATIONALE: A nurse should evaluate the efficacy of IV oxytocin therapy by assessing the uterine tone, monitoring vital signs, and getting a pad count. Assessing the skin turgor and assessing deep tendon reflexes are inappropriate interventions and are not applicable when administering oxytocin to the client.

CHAPTER 23

Activity A

1. Polycythemia
2. Gavage
3. asphyxia
4. preterm
5. atelectasis
6. term
7. Retinopathy
8. Pain
9. inversely
10. genetic

Activity B

1. **a.** The figure displays a low–birth-weight newborn in an Isolette.
   b. An Isolette keeps the newborn warm to conserve energy and prevent cold stress. The Isolette may be warmed or may have an overhead radiant warmer.

Activity C

1. c   2. a   3. b   4. d

Activity D

1.

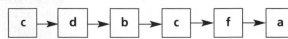

Activity E

1. The common physical characteristics of preterm newborns include
   • Birth weight of less than 5.5 lb
   • Scrawny appearance
   • Head disproportionately larger than chest circumference
   • Poor muscle tone
   • Minimal subcutaneous fat
   • Undescended testes
   • Plentiful lanugo (a soft downy hair), especially over the face and back
   • Poorly formed ear pinna with soft, pliable cartilage
   • Fused eyelids
   • Soft and spongy skull bones, especially along suture lines
   • Matted scalp hair, wooly in appearance
   • Absent or only a few creases in the soles and palms
   • Minimal scrotal rugae in male infants; prominent labia and clitoris in female infants
   • Thin, transparent skin with visible veins
   • Breast and nipples not clearly delineated
   • Abundant vernix caseosa

2. The clinical signs of hypoglycemia in the newborn are often subtle and include lethargy, apathy, drowsiness, irritability, tachypnea, weak cry, temperature instability, jitteriness, seizures, apnea, bradycardia, cyanosis or pallor, feeble suck and poor feeding, hypotonia, and coma. Blood glucose level below 40mg/dL in term newborns and below 20 mg/dL in preterm newborns is indicative of hypoglycemia in the newborn.

3. Developmentally supportive care is defined as care of a newborn or infant to support growth and development. Developmental care focuses on what newborns or infants can do at that stage of development; it uses therapeutic interventions only to the point that they are beneficial; and it provides for the development of the newborn–family unit.

4. Preterm infants are at a high risk for neurodevelopmental disorders such as cerebral palsy or mental retardation, intraventricular hemorrhage, congenital anomalies, neurosensory impairment, behavioral disadaptation, and chronic lung disease.

5. The characteristics of large-for-gestational-age newborns are
   • Large body; appears plump and full-faced
   • Increase in body size is proportional
   • Head circumference and body length in upper limits of intrauterine growth
   • Poor motor skills
   • Difficulty in regulating behavioral states
   • More difficult to arouse to a quiet alert state

6. Post-term newborns typically exhibit the following characteristics:
   • Dry, cracked, wrinkled skin
   • Long, thin extremities
   • Creases that cover the entire soles of the feet
   • Wide-eyed, alert expression
   • Abundant hair on scalp
   • Thin umbilical cord
   • Limited vernix and lanugo
   • Meconium-stained skin
   • Long nails

Activity F

1. a. A nurse can help the parents in the detachment process in the following ways:
  - To see their newborn through the maze of equipment
  - Explain the various procedures and equipment
  - Encourage them to express their feelings about the fragile newborn's status
  - Provide the parents time to spend with their dying newborn

b. The nursing interventions when caring for a family experiencing a perinatal loss are as follows:
  - Help the family to accept the reality of death by using the word "died"
  - Acknowledge their grief and the fact that their newborn has died
  - Help the family to work through their grief by validating and listening
  - Provide the family with realistic information about the causes of death
  - Offer condolences to the family in a sincere manner
  - Initiate spiritual comfort by calling the hospital clergy if needed
  - Acknowledge variations in spiritual needs and readiness
  - Encourage the parents to have a funeral or memorial service to bring closure
  - Encourage the parents to take photographs, make memory boxes, and record their thoughts in a journal
  - Suggest that the parents plant a tree or flowers to remember the infant
  - Explore with family members how they dealt with previous losses
  - Discuss meditation and relaxation techniques to reduce stress
  - Provide opportunities for the family to hold the newborn if they choose to do so
  - Assess the family's support network
  - Address attachment issues concerning subsequent pregnancies
  - Reassure the family that their feelings and grieving responses are normal
  - Provide information about local support groups
  - Provide nticipatory guidance regarding the grieving process
  - Recommend that family members maintain a healthy diet and get adequate rest and exercise to preserve their health

Activity G

1. Answer: a
RATIONALE: The nurse should focus on decreasing blood viscosity by increasing fluid volume in the newborn with polycythemia. Checking blood glucose within two hours of birth by a reagent test strip and screening every two to three hours or before feeds are not interventions that will alleviate the condition of an infant with polycythemia. The nurse should monitor and maintain blood glucose levels when caring for a newborn with hypoglycemia, not polycythemia.

2. Answer: a, c, & e
RATIONALE: To minimize the risk of infections, the nurse should avoid coming to work when ill, use sterile gloves for an invasive procedure, and monitor laboratory test results for changes. The nurse should remove all jewelry prior to washing hands, not cover the jewelry. The nurse should use disposable equipment rather than avoid it.

3. Answer: a
RATIONALE: When preterm infants receive sensorimotor interventions such as rocking, massaging, holding, or sleeping on waterbeds, they gain weight faster, progress in feeding abilities more quickly, and show improved interactive behavior. Interventions such as swaddling and positioning, use of minimal amount of tape, and use of distraction through objects are related to pain management.

4. Answer: c
RATIONALE: The nurse should identify acute respiratory complication as the risk to the newborn that results from meconium in the amniotic fluid. Bradycardia, perinatal asphyxia, and polycythemia are some of the common problems faced by an SGA newborn but are not related to meconium in the amniotic fluid.

5. Answer: d
RATIONALE: A good cry or good breathing efforts are signs that the resuscitation has been successful. A pulse above 100 bpm, not 80 bpm, is an indication of a successful resuscitation. Pink tongue, not blue, indicates a good oxygen supply to the brain. Tremors are associated with the signs of hypothermia; this is not a sign of successful resuscitation.

6. Answer: c
RATIONALE: The nurse should observe for clinical signs of cold stress, such as respiratory distress, central cyanosis, hypoglycemia, lethargy, weak cry, abdominal distention, apnea, bradycardia, and acidosis. The temperature of the radiant warmer should not be set at a fixed level and should be adjusted to the newborn's temperature. The nurse need not check the blood pressure of the infant every two hours. The infant's temperature should be measured more often than every five hours.

7. Answer: b
RATIONALE: The nurse should administer 0.5 to 1 mL/kg/h of breast milk enterally to induce surges in gut hormones that enhance maturation of the intestine. Administering vitamin D supplements, iron supplements, or intravenous dextrose will not significantly help the preterm newborn's gut overcome the many feeding difficulties.

8. Answer: a
RATIONALE: The nurse should maintain the fluid and electrolyte balance of an infant born with

hypoglycemia. Dextrose should be given intravenously only if the infant refuses oral feedings, not before offering the infant oral feedings. Placing the infant on a radiant warmer will not help maintain blood glucose levels. The nurse should focus on decreasing blood viscosity in an infant who is at risk for polycythemia, not hypoglycemia.

9. **Answer: c**
   RATIONALE: The nurse should assess for a decrease in urinary output and fluid balance in the preterm or post-term newborn. Weight of the newborn should be measured daily, not once every two days. Increased muscle tone does not indicate nutrition and fluid imbalance. A rise, not fall, in temperature indicates dehydration.

10. **Answer: a, b, & d**
    RATIONALE: Diabetes mellitus, postdates gestation, and glucose intolerance are the maternal factors the nurse should consider that could lead to a newborn being large for gestational age. Renal condition and maternal alcohol use are not factors associated with a newborn's being large for gestational age.

11. **Answer: a**
    RATIONALE: Jaundice is a sign of polycythemia. Restlessness, temperature instability, and wheezing are not fetal distress signs; they are the signs of a newborn with hypothermia.

12. **Answer: c**
    RATIONALE: The nurse should administer glucose intravenously to the newborn immediately when the blood glucose level is less than 23 mg/dL. Administering dextrose intravenously or placing the infant on a radiant warmer will not help maintain the glucose level. Monitoring the infant's pulse is not a priority.

13. **Answer: a, c, & e**
    RATIONALE: Hydration, early feedings, and phototherapy are measures that the nurse should take to reduce bilirubin levels in the newborn. Increasing the infant's water intake or administering vitamin supplements will not help reduce bilirubin levels in the infant.

14. **Answer: c**
    RATIONALE: A stained umbilical cord indicates a possibility of meconium aspiration, and the nurse should inform the primary care provider immediately. Listlessness or lethargy by themselves do not indicate meconium aspiration. Bluish skin discoloration is normal in infants, and so is pink discoloration of the tongue.

CHAPTER 24

Activity A

1. omphalocele
2. Cephalohematoma
3. Hyperbilirubinemia
4. sepsis
5. Methadone
6. hemolytic
7. phototherapy
8. Gastroschisis
9. asphyxia
10. Kernicterus
11. inflammatory
12. ventriculoperitoneal

Activity B

1. The congenital condition is known as esophageal atresia. It is the most common type of esophageal atresia in which the esophagus ends in a blind pouch and a fistula connects the trachea with the distal portion of the esophagus.

2. This equipment is a Pavlik harness. If the newborn exam reveals developmental dysplasia of the hip (DDH), the newborn is referred to an orthopedist. The goal of treatment is to relocate the femoral head in the acetabulum to facilitate normal growth and development. The Pavlik harness is the most widely used device; it prevents adduction while allowing flexion and abduction to accomplish the treatment goal.

Activity C

I.

1. a   2. d   3. b   4. c

II.

1. d   2. b   3. c   4. a

Activity D

1. The characteristics of infants born to diabetic mothers are:
   * Full rosy cheeks with a ruddy skin color
   * Short neck with a buffalo hump over the nape of the neck
   * Massive shoulders showing full intrascapular area
   * Distended upper abdomen due to organ overgrowth
   * Excessive subcutaneous fat tissue, producing fat extremities

2. The most common types of malformations in infants of diabetic mothers involve anomalies in the following systems:
   * Cardiovascular
   * Skeletal
   * Central nervous system
   * Gastrointestinal
   * Genitourinary

3. The treatment of infants born to diabetic mothers focuses on correcting hypoglycemia, hypocalcemia, hypomagnesemia, dehydration, and jaundice. Oxygenation and ventilation for the newborn are supported as necessary.

4. Birth trauma may result from the pressure of birth, especially in a prolonged or abrupt labor, abnormal or difficult presentation, cephalopelvic disproportion, or mechanical forces such as a forceps or vacuum used during delivery.

5. Meconium aspiration syndrome occurs when the newborn inhales particulate meconium mixed with amniotic fluid into the lungs while still in utero or on taking the first breath after birth. It is a common cause of newborn respiratory distress and can lead to severe illness.

6. Periventricular–intraventricular hemorrhage (PVH/IVH) is defined as bleeding that usually originates in the subependymal germinal matrix region of the brain, with extension into the ventricular system. It is a common problem of preterm infants, especially those born before 32 weeks.

7. Goals of therapy include restoring urinary continence, preserving renal function, and reconstructing functional and cosmetically acceptable genitalia.

8. Encourage the parents to express their feelings about this highly visible anomaly. Emphasize the newborn's positive features and role model nurturing behaviors when interacting with the infant. Encourage parental interaction and involvement with the newborn. Provide support to the parents, especially related to feeding difficulties. Allow them to vent their frustrations. Offer practical suggestions and continued encouragement for their efforts.

Activity E

1. The role of the nurse in handling substance-abusing mothers includes:
   - Being knowledgeable about issues of substance abuse
   - Being alert for opportunities to identify, prevent, manage, and educate clients and families about this key public health issue

2. The nurse can use the "5 A's" approach in the following way:
   - Ask: Ask the client if she smokes and if she would like to quit.
   - Advise: Encourage the use of clinically proved treatment plans.
   - Assess: Provide motivation by discussing the 5 R's:
     - Relevance of quitting to the client
     - Risk of continued smoking to the fetus
     - Rewards of quitting for both
     - Roadblocks to quitting
     - Repeat at every visit
   - Assist: Help the client to protect her fetus and newborn from the negative effects of smoking.
   - Arrange: Schedule follow-up visits to reinforce the client's commitment to quit.

Activity F

1. **Answer: d**
   RATIONALE: The nurse should assess for end-expiratory grunting, a barrel-shaped chest with an increased anterior-posterior (AP) chest diameter, prolonged tachypnea, progression from mild to severe respiratory distress, intercostal retractions, cyanosis, surfactant dysfunction, airway obstruc-

tion, hypoxia, and chemical pneumonitis with inflammation of pulmonary tissues in a newborn with meconium aspiration syndrome. A high-pitched cry may be noted in periventricular–intraventricular hemorrhage. Bile-stained emesis occurs in necrotizing enterocolitis. Increased intracranial pressure occurs in cases of hydrocephalus.

2. **Answer: a**
   RATIONALE: The nurse should assess for systolic ejection murmur. Respiratory alkalosis, rhinorrhea, and lacrimation may be symptoms of neonatal abstinence syndrome.

3. **Answer: d**
   RATIONALE: Noting any absence of or decrease in deep tendon reflexes is a nursing intervention when assessing a newborn with a risk for trauma. The nurse should examine the skin for cyanosis, should be alert for signs of apathy and listlessness, and should assess for any temperature instability when caring for a newborn born to a diabetic mother. These interventions are not required to assess for trauma or birth injuries in a newborn.

4. **Answer: b**
   RATIONALE: The nurse should know that the infant's mother must have been a diabetic. The large size of the infant born to a diabetic mother is secondary to exposure to high levels of maternal glucose crossing the placenta into the fetal circulation. Common problems among infants of diabetic mothers include macrosomia, RDS, birth trauma, hypoglycemia, hypocalcemia and hypomagnesemia, polycythemia, hyperbilirubinemia, and congenital anomalies. Listlessness is also a common symptom noted in these infants. Infants born to clients who have abused alcohol, infants who have experienced birth traumas, or infants whose mothers have had a low birth weight are not known to exhibit these particular characteristics, although these conditions do not produce very positive pregnancy outcomes.

5. **Answer: a, d & e**
   RATIONALE: A nurse should associate obstructive hydrocephalus, vision or hearing defects, and cerebral palsy with newborns having periventricular–intraventricular hemorrhage. Acid–base imbalances are a complication occurring during exchange transfusion for lowering serum bilirubin levels. Pneumonitis is a complication associated with esophageal atresia.

6. **Answer: c**
   RATIONALE: The nurse should assess for meconium aspiration syndrome in the newborn. Meconium aspiration involves patchy, fluffy infiltrates unevenly distributed throughout the lungs and marked hyperaeration mixed with areas of atelectasis that can be seen through chest x-rays. Direct visualization of the vocal cords for meconium staining using a laryngoscope can confirm aspiration. Lung auscultation typically reveals coarse

crackles and rhonchi. Arterial blood gas analysis will indicate metabolic acidosis with a low blood pH, decreased PaO2, and increased PaCO2. Newborns with choanal atresia, necrotizing enterocolitis, and hyperbilirubinemia are not known to exhibit these manifestations.

7. **Answer: a**

RATIONALE: The nurse should administer IV fluids and gavage feedings until the respiratory rate decreases enough to allow oral feedings when caring for a newborn with transient tachypnea. Maintaining adequate hydration and performing gentle suctioning are relevant nursing interventions when caring for a newborn with respiratory distress syndrome. The nurse need not monitor the newborn for signs and symptoms of hypotonia since hypotonia is not known to occur due to transient tachypnea. Hypotonia is observed in newborns with inborn errors of metabolism or in cases of preventricular-intraventricular hemorrhage.

8. **Answer: b**

RATIONALE: Ensuring effective resuscitation measures is the nursing intervention involved when treating a newborn for asphyxia. Ensuring adequate tissue perfusion and administering surfactant are nursing interventions involved in the care of newborns with meconium aspiration syndrome. Similarly, administering intravenous (IV) fluids is a nursing intervention involved in the care of newborns with transient tachypnea.

9. **Answer: c**

RATIONALE: The preoperative nursing care focuses on preventing aspiration by elevating the head of the bed 30 to 45 degrees to prevent reflux. Providing colostomy care is a part of postoperative nursing care for the newborn. Documenting the amount and color of drainage is the postoperative nursing care for a newborn with omphalocele. Administering antibiotics and total parenteral nutrition is a postoperative nursing intervention when caring for a newborn with esophageal atresia.

10. **Answer: d**

RATIONALE: When caring for a substance-exposed newborn, the nurse should check the newborn's skin turgor and fontanels. Encouraging early initiation of feedings and monitoring the newborn's cardiovascular status is a nursing intervention involved when caring for a newborn with pathologic jaundice. In cases of pathologic jaundice, the nurse also encourages supplementing breast milk with formula to supply protein if bilirubin levels continue to increase with breastfeeding only.

11. **Answer: b**

RATIONALE: The nurse should shield the newborn's eyes and cover the genitals to protect these areas from becoming irritated or burned when using direct lights and to ensure exposure of the greatest surface area. The nurse should place the newborn under the lights or on the fiberoptic blanket, exposing as much skin as possible. Breast or bottle feedings should be encouraged every two to three hours. Loose, green, and frequent stools indicate the presence of unconjugated bilirubin in the feces. This is normal; therefore, there is no need for therapy to be discontinued. Lack of frequent green stools is a cause for concern.

12. **Answer: b, d & e**

RATIONALE: When caring for a newborn with meconium aspiration syndrome, the nurse should place the newborn under a radiant warmer or in a warmed Isolette, administer oxygen therapy as ordered via a nasal cannula or with positive pressure ventilation, and administer broad-spectrum antibiotics to treat bacterial pneumonia. Repeated suctioning and stimulation should be limited to prevent overstimulation and further depression in the newborn. The nurse should also ensure minimal handling to reduce energy expenditure and oxygen consumption that could lead to further hypoxemia and acidosis. Handling and rubbing the newborn with a dry towel is needed to stimulate the onset of breathing in a newborn with asphyxia.

13. **Answer: a**

RATIONALE: The nurse should know that gastroschisis is a herniation of abdominal contents in which there is no peritoneal sac protecting herniated organs. A peritoneal sac is present in omphalocele. In gastroschisis, the herniated organs are not normal; they are unprotected and become thickened, edematous, and inflamed due to exposure to amniotic fluid. Gastroschisis is not a defect of the umbilical ring; it is a herniation of abdominal contents through an abdominal wall defect. Despite surgical correction, feeding intolerance, failure to thrive, and prolonged hospital stays occur in nearly all newborns with gastroschisis.

14. **Answer: c**

RATIONALE: The nurse should inform the parents that surgery for necrotizing enterocolitis requires the placement of a proximal enterostomy and ostomy care. Surgically treated NEC is a lengthy process and the amount of bowel that has necrosed, as determined during the bowel resection, significantly increases the likelihood that infants requiring surgery for NEC may have long-term medical problems. If surgery for NEC is required, antibiotics may be needed for an extended period of time.

15. **Answer: a**

RATIONALE: Bronchopulmonary dysplasia can be prevented by administering steroids to the mother in the antepartal period and exogenous surfactant to the newborn to aid in reducing the development of RDS and its severity. A high oxygen content can cause damage to the neonatal lung. Steroid injections for newborns at risk for BPD do not help the lungs mature. Giving exogenous surfactant to the mother does not increase the level of surfactant in the infant.

16. **Answer: b**
RATIONALE: After birth, carefully assess the newborn's cardiovascular and respiratory systems, looking for signs and symptoms of respiratory distress, cyanosis, or congestive heart failure that might indicate a cardiac anomaly. Assess rate, rhythm, and heart sounds, reporting any abnormalities immediately. Note any signs of heart failure, including edema, diminished peripheral pulses, hepatomegaly, tachycardia, diaphoresis, respiratory distress with tachypnea, peripheral pallor, and irritability (Kenner & Lott, 2007). Capillary refill time and the color of the infant's hands and feet are important to note but do not indicate possible heart failure. Neither does the blood glucose level.

17. **Answer: c**
RATIONALE: Provide comfort measures to the newborn who will be subjected to a variety of painful procedures. Be vigilant in ensuring the newborn's comfort, since he or she cannot report or describe pain. Assist in preventing pain as much as possible; interpret the newborn's cues suggesting pain and manage it appropriately.

18. **Answer: d**
RATIONALE: A myelomeningocele is a more severe form of spina bifida cystica, in which the spinal cord and nerve roots herniate into the sac through an opening in the spine, compromising the meninges. A meningocele includes the meninges and spinal fluid only. Spina bifida occulta is a defect in the vertebrae only. Spina bifida cystica is a generalized term that includes both a meningocele and a myelomeningocele.

19. **Answer: c**
RATIONALE: Measure head circumference daily to observe for hydrocephalus. Level of irritability is a much later sign of hydrocephalus in an infant. Weight and movement of the legs are not assessments that would indicate hydrocephalus.

20. **Answer: a, b & c**
RATIONALE: Administer prescribed medications as ordered. For example, give inotropics to support systemic blood pressure. Administer surfactant, steroids, and inhaled nitric oxide as ordered to correct hypoxia and acid–base imbalance.

21. **Answer: b**
RATIONALE: Repairing the facial anomaly as soon as possible is important to facilitate bonding between the newborn and the parents and to improve nutritional status. Treatment of cleft lip is surgical repair between the ages of 6 and 12 weeks.

22. **Answer: a**
RATIONALE: The degree of hypospadias depends on the location of the opening. It is often accompanied by a downward bowing of the penis (chordee), which can lead to urination and erection problems in adulthood. Prepuce is the foreskin of the penis. Priapism is an abnormally prolonged erection of the penis. Cholangi is a bile duct.

23. **Answer: d**
RATIONALE: Treatment for either type starts with serial casting, which is needed due to the rapid growth of the newborn. Surgery, braces, and physical therapy all have their place in the treatment of one or the other type of club foot, but they follow the initial treatment of serial casting.

24. **Answer: a**
RATIONALE: Ortolani's maneuver elicits the sensation of the dislocated hip reducing. Barlow's maneuver detects the hip dislocating from the acetabulum. Pavlik is a harness, not a maneuver. Bill's maneuver is an obstetric procedure of using forceps to turn the baby's head prior to birth.

25. **Answer: b, c & e**
RATIONALE: Retinopathy of the preterm newborn typically develops in both eyes secondary to an injury such as hyperoxemia due to prolonged assistive ventilation and high oxygen exposure, acidosis, and shock.